Reverence for All Life

The Path to Ahimsa

❖

VEGETARIANISM

JANICE GRAY KOLB

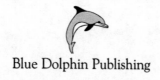

Blue Dolphin Publishing

Published by Blue Dolphin Publishing, Inc.
P.O. Box 8, Nevada City, CA 95959
Orders: 1-800-643-0765
Web: www.bluedolphinpublishing.com

ISBN: 978-1-57733-258-9 paperback
ISBN: 978-1-57733-436-1 e-book

Library of Congress Cataloging-in-Publication Data

Kolb, Janice E. M.
    Reverence for all life : the path to ahimsa : vegetarianism / Janice
Gray Kolb.
        p. cm.
    Includes bibliographical references.
    ISBN 978-1-57733-258-9 (pbk. : alk. paper)—
ISBN 978-1-57733-436-1 (e-book)
    1. Animal welfare—Religious aspects—Christianity.
    2. Vegetarianism—Religious aspects—Christianity. I. Title.
    BT746.K634 2012
    241'.693—dc23
                                                    2012012150

Photos and drawings by the Author

Cover photo of Moose taken by Author—as seen and written about in
author's books Beneath the Stars and Trees—There Is a Place and words
about moose and poem from A Pilgrim on Life's Road

A portion of any profits realized by sale of this book will be used to
support various animal charities.

Printed in the United States of America

10   9   8   7   6   5   4   3   2   1

Dedicated
to my
beloved feline
soulmate
Rochester

and

to my
beloved
husband and soulmate
Bob

Dear Father, hear and bless
Thy beasts and singing birds,
And guard with tenderness
Small things that have no words.

—Anonymous

I am the voice of the voiceless;
Through me the dumb will speak.
'Til the deaf world's ear be made to hear
The wrongs of the wordless weak.

And I am my brother's keeper,
And I will fight his fight;
And speak the word for beast and bird
'Til the world shall set things right.

—Ella Wheeler Wilcox (1850–1919)

Unseen they suffer
Unheard they cry—

"In the glance of the speechless animal there is a discourse
that only the soul of the wise can really understand."

—an Indian poet (from *The Treasury of Kahlil Gibran*)

Contents

We need another and a wiser and perhaps a more mystical concept of animals. We patronize them for their incompleteness, for their tragic fate of having taken form so far below ourselves. And therein we err, and greatly err. For the animal shall not be measured by man. In a world older and more complete than ours they move finished and complete, gifted with extensions of the senses we have lost or never attained, living by voices we shall never hear. They are not brethren, they are not underlings, they are other nations, caught with ourselves in the net of life and time, fellow prisoners of the splendour and travail of the earth.

—Henry Beston, from his book *The Outermost House,*
the enduring classic of a solitary year of life
in a small cottage on the Great Beach of Cape Cod

A Word in Preparation

OVER TWENTY YEARS AGO my wife Jan announced to me that she had decided to no longer eat meat, fish, or poultry. This was no complicated decision for her. She hadn't struggled and pondered this major decision. She simply decided that with her view and love of animals, it was no longer possible for her to eat them. Without a great deal of thought she made a vow to never again eat meat. She didn't ask me to make a similar vow or even push me hard to make that decision. She simply stopped. Not gradually or when we were alone, but full time. I am certain that to this day that vow has never been broken. For the next two or three months I watched her as she lived that vow. There was no stress or doubt related to her new eating habits, but peace and assuredness that she had made a proper decision. Slowly, and with no pressure exerted by her, I began to see the merit in her decision. I saw that her eating habits were healthy and provided proper nutritional support and balance. Without hardly recognizing it I was joining her and realized that weeks had passed without having one bit of meat, fish or poultry. I made no vow or even a promise to myself that I would not eat animal flesh, but I found that she was providing me with healthy nutritional meals that were delicious and satisfying. Now I have passed the twenty year mark of being a vegetarian and have no intention of changing. Over the years it has become increasingly easy to be a vegetarian. When we first made that decision, there were no meat substitutes available. Now the markets offer many products that mimic meat and are delicious. The list of available products now includes just about every meat taste I ate before, presented in such a way that I am now eating healthier more nutritious food.

When we sit down to eat, we now symbolically stand up for animals. We feel we are celebrating kindness and compassion and offering no support for the cruelty and misery that some animal farmers allow. If you are considering a vegetarian life, instead of thinking of what you will be missing, think instead about the new eating adventures you will experience. Many books offer delicious recipes and the internet provides literally thousands of ideas for vegetarian taste adventures.

For some people, making a quick decision like my wife Jan did, works well. For others it is a slow process, usually based on your own health and taste expectations—and a recognition of what actually happens to animals as they journey toward your plate. There are an increasing number of people who now become vegetarians one designated day of the week. Others have decided to never eat meat at home, but will accept a meat dinner at a restaurant because it is true that in many restaurants it is difficult to get a full meal that eliminates meat entirely.

The focus of the author in the pages that follow will be to convince you, for the sake of the animals, that vegetarianism is a good thing. If we would deeply involve our thinking as she has in what actually transpires along the road to put meat on our tables, most of us would respond with horror. But by remaining uninformed we can sit back comfortably and ignore reality. Let's try to look at ourselves and our culture from a non-personal position. We can then be more analytic about the situation and see what we have become. All it takes for this cruelty to animals to persist and prosper is for "nice guys" like us to just never think about it and the discomfort it would cause us if we did. If the physical and mental abuses were visited upon our pet cats and dogs to the same degree that they are forced upon animals destined for slaughter and for our appetites, the perpetrators would be prosecuted and severely punished. If I had taken a vow never to eat meat again, the problems of decision making would be gone. But because I have never made that vow, I force myself, whenever I contemplate eating meat, to actively think about the cruelty that is being forced upon some farm animals as they are fattened and prepared for our tables. The result is that I again make the "no meat" decision. I firmly believe that if done thoughtfully, a vegetarian life style is fully satisfying, fully healthy, and a strong statement of social concerns on how we should treat the animals we share this planet with.

—Robert A. Kolb Jr.

$\mathcal{A}$cknowledgments

*May the words of this book—and the meditation of our hearts
(the readers—and mine)—give glory to God
all glory to my Christ
and love and gratitude to Blessed Mother Mary
who always intercedes.*

I wish to thank my
Guardian Angel
and my special Angels
who are ever present.

I wish to express my deepest appreciation to Paul M. Clemens, publisher of Blue Dolphin Publishing, for believing in this book and for his kindness and grief support and to his capable staff who helped in so many ways. I especially thank Linda Maxwell for her fine work and friendship.

I wish to thank Rochester for his constant love, presence, devotion, inspiration, and teachings throughout our life together. Because of him this book was written.

I am deeply grateful to my husband Bob for his love and support, for believing in me, and for our life together in New Hampshire. I am grateful too for the time he gave in endless hours typing this manuscript.

I wish to thank
St. Francis of Assisi
and
St. Martin dePorres
for their great love and protection of all God's creatures.

The same force formed the sparrow
That fashioned man—the king
The God of the whole gave a living soul
To furred and to feathered thing.

—Ella Wheeler Wilcox from *Compassion
for All Creatures*, Janice Gray Kolb

"From an early age, I have abjured the use of meat,
and the time will come when men will look upon the murder of
animals as they look upon the murder of men."

—Leonardo DaVinci

"When we sit down to eat, we now symbolically stand up for
animals."

—Bob Kolb

Introduction

"Until he extends the circle of his compassion to all living things, man will not himself find peace."

—Albert Schweitzer from *Compassion for All Creatures,* Janice Gray Kolb)

WHEN THE IDEA OF THIS BOOK was first suggested to me by my publisher Paul M. Clemens, it was 2009. This was very significant to me that he should present these thoughts at that time, for it was then twenty years since my husband and I had become vegetarians. It seemed appropriate to now encourage others anew after we had been experiencing and living the vegetarian way of life for this length of time. We know and believe that this commitment was worthy and of God and that it is the time to bring forth again the events and inspiration that caused this major step. The overall and initial inspiration was from Rochester, my precious marmalade and white cat who entered my life in 1986. His mere presence and my deep love for him and he for me was the beginning of it all. I knew I had to take the path of vegetarianism and had already stopped eating meat years before, at least five years before Rochester came into my life. I was led to a book in 1989 that I will mention here in this book that then led me to my total commitment of no meat, fish or poultry ever again on my plate. And in 1997 my own book was published, *Compassion for All Creatures: An Inspirational*

Guide for Healing the Ostrich Syndrome. My handsome Rochester, inspiration for it all, is on the beautiful cover.

Now it is time to bring forth this basic message from *Compassion*, lifting it out from all related subjects I have written about in the book concerning respect and dignity for animals which includes non-killing and all other violence toward them. It is time to address this anew, for animals are still being horrendously treated, abused, tortured and killed so that humans may have their dead bodies on their tables to consume daily. It may seem strange to some to incorporate into these thoughts in this introduction the symbol of AA.

I could never ever eat any creature even if my own survival and life depended on it, or if ridiculed or argued against. It is like AA in a sense—for one makes a commitment, a very serious and deep commitment to never again drink alcohol. To make a deliberate slip to just have one can send you spiraling down or into what was "before" in your very troubled life. Both are deep spiritual commitments. One is to save your own life and the other to save the lives of living creatures—and like the first in regard to alcohol, you will change your spiritual and physical life if you become a vegetarian—or a vegan. People attend daily AA meetings to feel that commitment and strength through fellow members, and talk and share about their own personal abstinence. One can also apply the letters of AA to "Animals Anonymous" and abstain from eating their flesh and bodies with a deep commitment not to ever do so for their sake and your own.

Bob and I are the only total vegetarians in our large family and we are our own support group. But with my deep love for my Rochester and all animals I could never slip. It is a sacred vow to God on my part and to Rochester.

It is no casual comparison that has been made in regard to vegetarianism and alcohol, for Bob and I have attended many AA meetings in the past two years both in New Hampshire and

Pennsylvania. We do not drink alcohol at all and it has never been a part of our life. We raised our six children in this way. However, each individual is their own person and leads their own life and so alcohol made its way into our very large family and terribly affected one person. In order to give deepest love and support to someone we deeply love we then began to attend AA meetings with this loved one whenever we had the blessings of the three of us being together in either state. I can say that I feel we learned more than can be imagined from these meetings and felt privileged to be at each one we attended. We will continue to attend them whenever our presence is desired by our loved one or even otherwise. The books and material I own and read from AA are inspiring and strengthening. Applied to the non-eating of the flesh and bodies of animals, one can certainly see the similarity and need for commitment.

I have numerous times had an example thrown out at me concerning things that happened in real life and reported in books and on the news. What if one was in a plane crash, stranded in freezing temperatures, as was a true life situation, and one was dying of starvation? What then? Would you not eat the flesh of a companion traveller who did not survive so that you may have life? I am sure there are various answers. I have been told several. But I can write here that that surely is a situation that does not leave me in indecision. I emphatically would never ever consume another being in order that I might live. Ever! I would choose death and pass on like the others. There is a certain line that can never be crossed if one is a spiritual being. God sees and knows.

And for me, eating the flesh and bodies of dear animals is exactly the same as the example regarding a human I have just presented, no matter what the situation. Except in this case of the consumption of animals there are healthy and wonderful alternative choices to make of fruits and vegetables and delicious meals created from these gifts from God. You will not find recipes in this book for creating such meals, but you will learn about creating a heart and mind of compassion. One can live a healthy life with scrumptious and satisfying meals and good energy, and allow all God's creatures to live their lives also.

I pray that in continuing to read these pages you will find inspiration and strength and courage to begin a life of vegetarianism if you are indeed already not doing so now. It truly is a precious path to follow—that of *Ahimsa*.

Janice Gray Kolb
Higher Ground on Lake Balch
East Wakefield, New Hampshire

Introduction from Compassion for All Creatures

I introduce you now to the Introduction that appears in my book *Compassion for All Creatures* with only one paragraph omitted that is very informative but does not pertain to vegetarianism

"One does not meet oneself until one catches the reflection from an eye other than human."

—Loren Eiseley

FOR MANY YEARS NOW I have been experiencing a very extraordinary truth. The closer that one comes to God and the longer one spends in His Presence in quiet and solitude—wordlessly just enjoying His Friendship and Love—the more one is filled with deepening compassion. People and situations that once did not catch my attention, even though I have always tried to be very caring, now most certainly do have my involvement and help in ways that He leads. He seems to send many to me—even strangers—and they do not seem to be strangers when we encounter. Tears well up at the strangest times when I am alone just merely thinking of a sadness or wound that someone is bearing, and in conversation with some I find the tears there also as we share deeply in Spirit or speak of others who need our help. The tears just spill out without warning—because He has put this unexplainable compassion within me—just as He has put it in the hearts of others. The outrageous accounts of suffering heard and seen on the news leave imprints on me and memories of them I cannot shake. I pray! War is horrifying to me—that humans are killing each other and innocent children and others are slain in horrendous ways.

But when God places His deep compassion in a heart, it is not only for human beings—at least I have found this to be so. In recent years my compassion for all God's creatures has increased to dimensions I never thought possible. I cannot bear to hear of any cruelty to any creature no matter how large or how small. Animals and other living species—like the unborn of humans that are often senselessly aborted—have no voice. They are often tortured and killed mercilessly as if they are incapable of pain. I am one of many who feel this is extremely wrong, and who wants to be their voice.

In the past few years a deep impression was put upon my heart to write about God's creatures and to look at them in ways perhaps many have not considered. I know this impression came from His Spirit, for I have known such calls before and followed.

In the pages of this book are deep personal sharings from my own life in regard to animals and also many true accounts of the experiences of others. There are truths to consider and reflect upon that you may not have known before and there is scripture to ponder in relation to animals. It is a book mainly written for Christians, but is essentially for any one who wishes to take a new look at the creatures God placed into our care and to search his or her own heart in their regard.

Though I have loved many animals personally, there is one little feline in particular who has changed my life. I know he was given to me by the One who put these stirrings within me that would not leave—the stirrings that caused the writing of this book.

Those who know me well know that when I love—I LOVE—and so perhaps you who do not know me may find personal sharings of my relationship with my little cat quite unusual. But I have learned there are many like myself that will not find me "too strange" through the confessions I have made and the happenings in my life that I have been led to write down for all to see.

Living in the woods amongst nature on the shore of a lake has changed the way my husband and I view life. Wild little creatures come up on our porch and peer through our sliding glass doors and my little cat and they respond to each other through the screens or the glass. We have learned how intelligent these little beings are. We have seen them too outwit us and been amazed. We have watched the interchange between birds and squirrels and chipmunks all feeding at the same bird feeders at the same moments. We have been surprised and overwhelmed by families of raccoons silently observing us through the glass, patiently waiting to search our faces and responses. We have watched the beautiful herons land in our cove and the families of ducks waddle up our beach to wait for us to feed them—so trustingly. Too, we have heard the incredible wail of the loons in day and night and observed them dive for food into the lake or run across the water. Nothing can compare to the lapping water and wail of the loon in the night.

The beaver has managed to stay out of sight but he has freely let us know he is very much present. Though we have never seen one, we have been incredulous at the evidences of their close existence to us. I have pictures of raccoons hanging over our highest bird feeder at night, feasting well and with eyes gleaming red in the dark. I record the wild life with my camera as well as in keeping a wild life log in a journal placed by the window with binoculars. There are foxes and opossum and rabbits in the woods, and deer and moose not often seen. There are osprey and mallard ducks and other birds in large migratory groups.

And in Spring and early Summer when we open our windows, there is a most supernatural harmony that is heard at twilight and throughout evening until almost dawn that I have termed "Nightsong." It is as if every animal, bird and insect has joined voices and this celebration is so incredibly beautiful and awesome to hear in the dark before sleep—or if one wakes in the night. I somehow envision shafts of moonlight shining down through the trees into the woods and this dear Creature Choir all assembled in the grasses and branches and on rocks and directed by Snow White or a lovely Fairy Princess.

I put my watch aside and tell time by the sun going across the sky as I write at my desk, and night after night see God's sunsets on the lake. They never cease to inspire and leave me in awe and almost daily I take pictures as the sun goes down. According to season the color varies—and pink, orange and red sunsets throughout the year continue to cast their spell of magical color over heaven and lake's surface and woods and myself.

Living enfolded in Nature in all seasons of the year (for after this book was completed in 1997, we moved here permanently to the woods) gives one a new perspective. The earth and trees and God's creatures are part of us and I would not now even kill a bug or ant. If they are found inside, they are carried outdoors carefully. My husband has built a pro-life mouse trap, and if a little mouse enters it, tempted by the offering of jelly bean or peanut butter within, then he is caught. The trap looks like a little house and I have decorated the outside to look like a home at my husband's request. After greeting the little mouse within, he is taken outside in his house and the door is opened and he is set free. Perhaps he runs right back into our cottage, we cannot be sure. But it really does not matter. He will find his way into the Mouse House once more. (See Janice Gray Kolb, *The Astonishing Adventures of Luki Tawdry*, Papillon Publishing, 2012.) Life is good here and I have come to realize that each life, no matter how insignificant it appears to human beings, IS A LIFE. I cannot kill. We live in peace and harmony here and we let all else live in the same way.

There was a word that was not familiar to me until shortly before I began to write about God's creatures and was involved in reading about them concerning their treatment by the various religions of our world. I learned the word *"Ahimsa,"* which means "harmlessness" or not hurting, and that it is a Sanskrit word for "compassion." Wherever Ahimsa is found, there is deep compassion and unselfishness and service to others and a refraining from causing pain and suffering to any living creature. It naturally implies non-killing. In the numerous books in which I came upon the true meaning of this word, I also learned in each that to not cause injury truly means total abstinence from causing ANY harm or pain whatsoever to ANY living creature, either by thought, word or deed. It is LOVE! Universal Love! Long ago it was said that Ahimsa was prescribed by very wise men to eliminate cruel and brutal tendencies in man.

Ahimsa is said to be the highest and noblest of traits. To sum up all that Ahimsa is—is to learn that Ahimsa or non-violence has proven to be a great and mighty Spiritual force.

It is a trait that most surely we would desire in all religions. It is a word and subject that must be brought forth here to reflect upon as one continues now to read this book. It is a word and a teaching that I find essential to my life as a Christian and one that will remain with me as I strive to live it out. Its influence only deepens, and it is firmly entrenched in the compassion that Our Lord placed within my heart for humans and animals alike.

Please prayerfully investigate further and allow His Light to penetrate your mind and heart as you read—the same Light that brought all of this to light in my soul and caused me to investigate also—and then to write down all that I was shown and all the personal joys I have been experiencing since sharing my life with one of His furry little children.

These writings have been covered with prayer from beginning to end, and I personally pray that the Holy Spirit will guide you lovingly through the reading of them just as He guided me through the writing.

J.G.K.
Higher Ground on Lake Balch
E. Wakefield, New Hampshire

CHAPTER 1

When Love Came Down

*"Friendship is a union of spirits, a marriage of hearts,
and the bond thereof virtue."*

—William Penn

ON JUNE 23, 1986 Our Lord placed a gift down for me on a bench in a small mall in Rochester, New Hampshire. I did not know this gift was to be bestowed on me that day or on any day of my life, for this particular gift was one I had been forbidden to have for thirty-two years. Therefore, when it was placed there in a carton and all obstacles were removed from my being permitted to accept it, I was able to receive this gift with great inexpressible joy. A few years later words still cannot convey the depth of that joy that this gift has brought into my life. Only those who have been given a similar gift at some point in their lives can truly understand, and yet not quite so, for each gift is so utterly unique.

I was given a gift of love that warm June morning in the form of a tiny marmalade and white furry kitten approximately eight weeks old. He was free, as is our Lord's love. All we need to do is accept His love. And so I accepted that indescribable gift of love, and in doing so I have felt the Lord's love to me more vividly with every passing day.

Who could have known my life would be changed so by the acceptance of this unexpected gift! In His perfect timing He brought me to that very spot in the mall to receive His love in a new way. There is a beautiful quotation by an unknown author that has come to mind again and again since this wonderful creature has become my inseparable companion.

> God never loved me in so sweet a way before. 'Tis He alone who can such blessings send. And when His love would new expressions find, He brought thee to me and He said—Behold a friend.

This is what our Lord had done for me! I am eternally grateful and just as I am incapable of truly expressing the joy I feel, neither can I truly express my gratitude. I plead daily to Him to look into my heart and there He will find the joy and the gratitude bubbling over. He knows. It is written that "Our deepest feelings live in words unspoken."

I cannot now ever imagine my life without Rochester. Yes, Rochester. He is named for the town in which I received him and adopted him, and I felt it might possibly be the town in which he was born. Affectionately he is also known by the shortened version of his name, "Chester."

And so life is different now. Life is changed. A beautiful creature of God lives with me, sleeps with me and spends the majority of his hours near me or on my lap, and my life is enriched because of him. I see with new spiritual eyes matters I did not see vividly and with my whole heart before. He has changed my husband's life and other lives of my friends, and I can no longer keep all of this to myself. One small cat has turned my existence upside down and caused me to reflect on numerous things that before June 23, 1986 were not foremost in my thinking. I had to be gently shown in love, and daily educated by a most unusual teacher in order for my attention to be drawn more and more in this direction. And it has been a Christian education.

Let me tell you what I have been taught in this "School of Love" by Rochester. But first let me share with you the details of this adoption and our first days together.

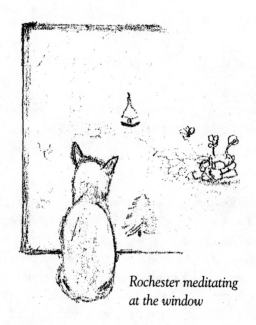

*Rochester meditating
at the window*

CHAPTER 2

❧

We Meet and the Angels Sing!

"I love these little people: and it is not a slight thing when they, who are so fresh from God, love us."

—Charles Dickens

THE BLACK AND WHITE VAN pulled into the very large parking lot of a very ordinary little mall in Rochester, New Hampshire. It was late morning of a bright and beautiful day in June and my husband and I smiled and commented on the blessing of our safe arrival. We slowly opened the doors, slid down from our seats and out of the van. Our teenage daughter, Janna, rolled gracefully out from the side door with her curly hair going in various directions and her expression still one of drowsiness. We had travelled through the night from our home in Pennsylvania and this stop was only to quickly buy groceries. We would take them with us to our cottage on Lake Balch some twenty-five miles further north.

As we entered the mall we were immediately confronted with a father and two children sitting on a round bench outside the supermarket and holding a sign that read "Free Kittens." Next to them on the bench was a closed carton. My daughter and I, upon encountering this sight, widened our eyes in a spontaneous secret signal to each other without my husband realizing what was about to befall him.

Now, lest you begin to feel sorry for my husband, let me hurriedly take you back many years in order to understand the scene that has been unravelling before your eyes. I had been born into a home with a cat and had grown up with cats. Until I married and left home exactly upon turning twenty-one, I had had the joy and companionship of cats. But the day I married Bob, he said emphatically, "No Cats!"

In my thirty-two years of marriage I had loved and reared six children—five wonderful daughters and a fine son. I had also loved and cared for three hardy and adorable little Cairn Terriers and all the puppies of their many litters. This also included a vacation when we travelled to New Hampshire with nine dogs and five children and an infant girl. One of the dogs had had six puppies the night before we were to leave and so they too had to vacation with us so that they might be close to their mother and be properly nourished.

There had also been hamsters during those thirty-two years, and guinea pigs, mice, turtles, gerbils, fish, and one hermit crab that was lost in our home.

All of these, but my husband had said, "No Cats!"

Occasionally throughout these many years I had asked if I might have a kitten. More recently our daughter Janna had voiced the same request. Always the answer came back—"No Cats!"

Ah, but this day in the mall in New Hampshire some supernatural power took over within me as I made my first pleas to Bob in order that Janna and I might have one of these free kittens. When his usual reply came back to me accompanied by the expression on his face I well recognized, I would not be silenced! I asked again. Again. AGAIN. I began to frighten myself in my persistence that refused to buckle under his rising anger and stormy appearance. I could not quiet my pleas until I at last, after thirty-two years, had won my simple request. Nothing else mattered in those moments but a "yes." I could never again bear to hear "No Cats!"

"All right, all right, get one, but I'll have nothing to do with it," he hissed. I began to say a continuous stream of "thank yous" and ran off to find my daughter who had delicately removed herself earlier from the muffled battle scene. Oh, the joy and excitement of the two of us as we stifled squeals of victory between us there in the aisle of the supermarket.

I, delirious with happiness, told my daughter to quickly go and pick out a kitten before her father changed his mind. I then dashed about the store to complete the shopping in a flash with the hope of assuaging Bob's anger by my promptness. Continuing our trip at once I felt would calm him.

Janna rushed back to find me. "Male or female?" she said.

"Female, I suppose, perhaps easier to train."

"But the little boy is so cute" said Janna. "He likes me!"

"Get the boy then quickly," I had said, and I finished the shopping with a final toss of kitty litter and cans of cat food into the basket.

I pushed the cart of groceries to the van and waiting husband, and Janna carried a carton. Peeking out whenever he could push his tiny head through was a beautiful pale orange and white kitten. Oh, I was ecstatic! Somehow I had expected to see a black cat like my cats had been years ago, and so the lovely light fur of this new kitten surprised me! He was perfect! My daughter sat in the seat behind, holding the carton as we drove, and the tiny face would pop out and look around. "I won't have a cat that is not clean!" stormed Bob. We drove further with Janna and I sneaking glances at each other while adoring the kitten. "I don't want to have to listen to a lot of meowing!" Bob said, as we drove further. "This cat will be nothing but trouble!" he continued, "And what will we do with him when we travel?"

Silence took over for a bit and then I suggested we give our sweet kitten a name. After several were thrown about to digest, it struck me that "Rochester" would be a fine name—after the town in which we had adopted him. It was voted a yes! Suddenly the man said, "Call him Chester for short." My daughter and I agreed and, exchanging glances, made no comment that her father had temporarily softened and joined in our joy. Once in our cottage and the litter box was prepared—the tiny Chester jumped in to test it, thereby setting a pattern of faithfulness. From that moment on he never gave Bob cause to accuse him of uncleanliness. He never made a mistake.

Soon we realized we had a very silent new family member, for Rochester never meowed. He spoke only from that day forward with his big loving golden eyes that matched his fur, and he padded and ran about softly on his little white marshmallow paws. He was so grateful to be ours! He would never be trouble! He obviously wanted Janna and me to be proud of him and he never gave cause for the man to be angry.

Each evening this dear little cat curled up on me as I slept, finding warm and comfortable places upon me to sleep throughout the night. One morning upon awakening I saw my kitten lying across the forehead of my husband as he laid on his back beneath the covers. I said nothing of this but spoke to Bob as if a kitten was not upon his forehead. He replied in like manner as I left the room. How hysterical it was to talk to him with Rochester on his face! I ran to the next room and burst into laughter! It was better left alone and unremarked upon. I did not want to make Bob feel foolish and I was so anxious that they come to know each other. This scene was often repeated from that day on.

As the days passed in the little cottage and Chester gave and gave his love to his new family, Janna and I soon began to hear:

"Hi, Harry!"

"Is your dinner good, Harry?"

"Where's Harry?"

Not able to express it, my husband had given our little cat another name, his secret way, perhaps even surprising and unexplainable to Bob himself, of showing a special affection for the tiny kitten. And oh how Chester proved he could travel and was not trouble to this man! In the first year of his life alone Rochester made fifteen trips from New Hampshire to Pennsylvania and back, travelling the entire ten hours each trip on my lap.

All the words in the world that my daughter and I could have searched for to try to convince Bob to accept the kitten were now not needed. The clean, obedient little Chester with his gift of continual silence and unconditional love had warmed Bob's heart and won for "Harry" his own acceptance.

❖

CHAPTER 3

Do Unto Others

*"There is no religion without love, and people may talk as much as
they like about their religion but if it does not teach them to be good
and kind
to other animals as well as humans, it is all a sham."*
—Anna Sewell, *Black Beauty*

Since Rochester has come to live with me and be my companion, there are many things that leave me appalled. His coming into my life has changed my life so drastically that I see this world and man in a new way. I can no longer live in the same manner in which I have in the past in regard to animals. Though I have always had a love for animals and many have inhabited our home, my eyes were not opened to things as I see them now until experiencing this deeper relationship with Rochester. It did not take long either before that change came to be, and every day it becomes more ingrained in me so that I could never ever be as I was before.

Gandhi has said in *An Autobiography: The Story of My Experiments:*

> To my mind the life of the lamb is no less precious than
> that of a human being. I should be unwilling to take the life of
> the lamb for the sake of the human body. I hold that, the more

helpless a creature, the more entitled it is to protection by man from the cruelty of man.

There are devout Christians I know well who cannot comprehend that an animal can be a fit and loving companion and in some cases a person's only companion and that it is a fulfilling relationship for this human who loves his companion so. I have seen shock and some disdain and disbelief when prayer is mentioned or given for an animal, and the disdain comes from Christians who have reputations for deep prayer lives. Why are Christians different from those of other faiths and religions in this way? And how can it continue if we expect to be witnesses to the world? I have heard Christians say, "I hate animals" and then laugh and think it is amusing.

I have tears within and feel deeply troubled when from the altars of churches, pastors and priests announce a ham-and-bean dinner for their parishioners to be served in the church halls. I have heard and witnessed such announcements—one just two weeks ago—and it saddened me that all these Christians after attending Mass—and feeding upon the Eucharist, Our Lord's Body and Blood—would go below with their pastor and feed on the dead bodies of many pigs. These many pigs had to be slaughtered in order for this large group to have an evening of sociability and fun when the same fellowship could be achieved without the suffering and slaughter of those animals. If one would read about pigs and learn of their intelligence and what they endure and suffer before the actual horrendous slaughter itself, then one could never eat a pig again.

Naturalist W.H. Hudson, in *Book of a Naturalist* (as quoted in John Robbins' *Diet for a New America)*, has said:

> I have a friendly feeling towards pigs and consider them the most intelligent of beasts. I also like his attitudes towards all other creatures, especially man. He views us from a totally different, a sort of democratic standpoint as fellow citizens and brothers, and takes for granted, or grunted, that we un-

derstand his language, and without servility or insolence he has a natural, pleasant, camaraderie—or hail-fellow-well-met air with us.

My husband, whose soul has been enlightened concerning the animals and eats now in this different way, even slows down and brakes for the tiny chipmunks that run into these country roads. It happened spontaneously and it gives us such joy to know that little lives are spared. He never harmed animals before, but now he is more aware and seeks to be especially cautious.

J.Todd Ferrier (1855-1943), in *On Behalf of Christians*, states:

> Western civilization, in seeking to conquer the east, has too often materialized the faith. And the failure of missionaries to win over the cultured of the east is through our gross western habits in living. For the man whose religion teaches him to hold all life sacred, is not likely to be converted to a faith that deems no life sacred but man's.

He continues, in *The Extended Circle: A Commonplace Book of Animal Rights*, to say:

> Much of the indifference, apathy, and even cruelty which we see has its origin in the false education given the young concerning the rights of animals and their duty towards them. It ought to make all who profess evangelical Christianity ashamed that the finest and most compassionate souls have not been within their own borders, but rather amongst those whose deepest thoughts have aroused the suspicion of heresy. Evangelical Christianity, as people understand it, has absolutely failed to kindle the Divine Compassion, and to realize itself in a great fire of sacred *devotion to all life*.

My Rochester is always a channel for God's love to others and "an instrument of Peace," a phrase the great animal lover, St. Francis of Assisi, used in his well-known prayer. Read this prayer now for the first time or read it anew, but read it perhaps for the first time in light of your relationship to God's wonderful creatures that share the world with us and what you personally may possibly be able to do for them.

The Prayer of Saint Francis

Lord, make me an instrument of Thy peace; Where there is hatred, let me sow love; Where there is doubt, faith; Where there is despair, hope; Where there is darkness, light, and where there is sadness, joy.

O Divine Master, grant that I may not so much seek to be consoled as to console; to be understood, as to understand; to be loved, as to love; for it is in giving that we receive, it is in pardoning that we are pardoned, and it is in dying that we are born to eternal life.

—St. Francis of Assisi

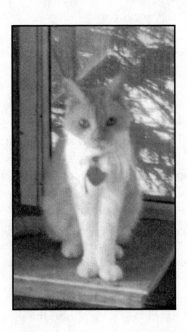

CHAPTER 4

$\mathcal{V}egetarianism$

"Animals are my friends and I don't eat my friends"
—George Bernard Shaw

OUR LORD has always used books in my life to lead me along in my spiritual journey. I have been an avid reader since I was a child and therefore it would seem that He chose the love of reading that was close to my heart to draw me more deeply into His Own Heart. Conversions and turning points in my existence were always associated with some book or books, and in reminiscing are naturally connected to these events most firmly. It was not strange then that I was led to make my commitment to vegetarianism through the finding and reading of a book, all within a short period of several days.

But before I write of this in detail I want to say that, since my change and enlightenment through a precious little cat, I often have pain and tears over the things in my past that did not show love to my fellow creatures. I grew up eating meat, poultry and fish and meals centered around these creatures. I never knew a vegetarian. All my friends grew up in the same way. I am guilty of raising my own family as I was raised, with the usual hamburger, chicken, turkey, occasional roasts and less seldom, fish. Like millions of Americans and Christians I made the carcass of a dead animal or bird the centerpiece of a festive meal. I did not know then what I know now. The Holy Spirit simply had not spoken to me about this—or I had not listened.

There was a slight breakthrough in the very early 1980s when I gave up red meat one Lenten period and never returned to eating it again. But I continued to eat other creatures and serve them to others. Then came the Macrobiotic Cooking Lessons in 1983. Our Lord used these cooking lessons to teach me about creatures, and also to learn that nutrition could be sound with a vegetarian life style. He also used the lessons to help me help my husband Bob as he awaited lung surgery in 1984 and to help my Peruvian friend who had cancer. And now I have met many vegetarians. They came to these cooking lessons—some by choice as a preventative and some because they were trying to heal themselves of cancer or addictions or other illnesses through this ancient Japanese diet. And I met the teacher and counsellors associated with the Macrobiotic Center.

Following these lessons and the using of less and less poultry and no red meat at all in cooking for my family, I found it disgusting to see chicken parts or handle them in order to prepare them. Even my two youngest daughters who often helped me cook were experiencing these same feelings. I no longer could prepare a turkey and found it terrible to see one as the center of attention at Thanksgiving in the home of one of my daughters who so lovingly had begun to take over my job of having our large family for dinner. But I could never say anything to hurt her, and the first Thanksgiving I was a vegetarian she did not even know it for I said nothing. I had found myself feeling such guilt each time I ate turkey or chicken since the Macrobiotic Cooking Lessons that I had rarely eaten any and it had come to be accepted and not particularly noticed one way or the other.

As the next Thanksgiving approached and this matter of the killing of so many turkeys was in the newspaper and I could envision the sadness of this slaughter and the resulting centerpiece at my own approaching family dinner, I wrote this poem one evening in mild protest and in love for these birds.

WHAT A BEAUTIFUL BIRD?!

O right before our very eyes—
Lies a turkey in demise.
He's there on platter—without head
And all will feed upon the dead.

Now a centerpiece—how odd—
When once he ran about the sod!
All stomachs become graveyards now—
And mashed potatoes bury fowl!

I dedicated it to "*All Turkeys.*" My deep bonding with Rochester continued to cause the guilt to be unbearable if I did give in to be polite and I ate poultry. To finally make the spiritual commitment to be a vegetarian was a joy and a relief. It was taken out of my hands from that moment on. I could never go back—it was irrevocable! And the decision and commitment has only intensified my love for animals and all creatures of air or water—and to feel pain at the inhuman treatment toward them. These feelings will only increase. I just pray that in some way, besides my prayers, my commitment will be a form of repentance in my life for all the years I was not enlightened—and though not directly ever killing an animal, I ate meat and poultry and fish killed by others. There is no way I can tell you what the animals suffer so that human beings—and millions of them Christians—can have what they feel is a necessity in their diets.

The Animal Rights Maxim is "*Do not eat anything with a face,*" and from that incredible thought and directive I wrote this little verse one evening.

An excellent rule for the human race—
When sitting down at its dinner place—
To alleviate pain—and death erase
Do not eat anything with a face.

Ralph Waldo Emerson (1803–1882) wrote:

> You have just dined, and however scrupulously the slaughter house is concealed in the graceful distance of miles, there is complicity.

And one can stew it, bake it, broil it, cover it with elegant sauces and fine gravies, but it is still a dead carcass one has prepared and put in the center of the table. In an essay "On Eating Flesh," an excerpt of which left its impact on my heart from the first reading, the Roman author Plutarch ended this essay describing the utter torment and torture and final slow slaughter of the animals with these words:

> for the sake of a little flesh we deprive them of sun, of light, of the duration of life to which they are entitled by birth and being.

He then delivered this challenge to flesh eaters:

> If you declare that you are naturally designed for such a diet, then first kill for yourself what you want to eat. Do it, however, only through your own resource unaided by cleaver or cudgel or any kind of ax.

The great Renaissance painter, inventor, sculptor and poet, Leonardo DaVinci, said: "He who does not value life does not deserve it."

He considered bodies of meat eaters to be "burial places"—grave yards for the animals they eat, and it was his thoughts read previous to my commitment that somewhat inspired the poem I wrote. His journals were filled with passages on compassion for animals. He also wrote:

> Endless numbers of these animals shall have their little children taken from them, ripped open, and barbarously slaughtered.

A Nonviolent Diet

It has been noted by not only the famous such as French philosopher Jean-Jacques Rousseau but by more recent studies by people involved in Macrobiotic Counselling and Cooking that many meat eaters tend to be more angry and volatile and that our diets do indeed affect our nature and temperament. "We are what we eat" is a well-known saying, and if people would read and study more how food affects human beings, they would be very surprised at the findings. It is known that women through their cooking can make their husbands more relaxed, docile and laid back. In our own home there was evidence of this both in my husband's temperament and my own reaction to eating simple brown rice alone for an extended period. There was a definite change in my husband and any evidence of a short temper disappeared and he was indeed a happier man. I became so relaxed and content to be absolutely still and contemplative that I had to force myself to do other things. This was an experiment we both tried—living on only short grain brown rice for ten days as written about in a famous book on Macrobiotic teaching. We later added vegetables and beans and other nourishing ingredients of the Macrobiotic Diet, but the original ten-day period of eating only short grain organic brown rice was a period of cleansing for the body. It is not harmful—in fact quite the opposite—and Monks in Japan and other Eastern countries are known to live on brown rice. It is the highest food. It truly does make one gentle and compassionate. Yellow-robed Buddhist Monks usually go barefoot and carry begging bowls. Besides robe and bowl a Monk owns little else. Other possessions are a needle, a string of 108 beads which he counts as he meditates on the qualities of Buddha, a razor with which to shave his head and a filter with which to strain insects from his drinking water so he will do them no harm. If even the insects are protected and cared for, his reverence for life is evident.

Other Vegetarians of Note

So many great men of the past were advocates of natural order and were vegetarians. Pythagoras, famous for contributions to geometry and mathematics, was an example to many who followed thereafter. He ate only herbs and vegetables and honey and it was written he would also pay fishermen to throw their catch back into the sea. Those who followed his teachings were DaVinci, Rousseau, Benjamin Franklin, the poet Shelley and his wife and many others. Benjamin Franklin became a vegetarian at age sixteen and called flesh eating "unprovoked murder" in his autobiographical writings. Unfortunately many years later he was persuaded to return to the eating of fish.

Russian author Leo Tolstoy advocated "vegetarian pacifism" after a total life change and never killed anything, not even an ant. He felt that in violence there was a natural progression that led to war in human society. He felt flesh eating "immoral."

Composer Richard Wagner also believed all life was sacred. He felt vegetarianism could save mankind from violent tendencies. Henry David Thoreau was a vegetarian at various periods in his life and though he at times wavered—but returned to the diet—he recognized its virtues. He wrote in Walden:

> Is it not a reproach that man is a carnivorous animal? True, he can and does live in great measure, by preying on other animals, but this is a miserable way—as any one who will go to snaring rabbits, or slaughtering lambs, may learn—and he will be regarded as a benefactor of his race who shall teach man to confine himself to a more innocent and wholesome diet. Whatever my own practice may be, I have no doubt that it is a part of the destiny of the human race, in its gradual improvement, to leave off eating animals, as surely as the savage tribes have left off eating each other when they came in contact with the more civilized.

Mahatma Gandhi is perhaps the one most known for this way of "ahimsa" (or non-violence) and vegetarian diet. He stated:

> I do feel that spiritual progress does demand at some stage that we should cease to kill our fellow creatures for the satisfaction of our bodily wants.

He founded Tolstoy Farm where vegetarian principles were the basis for this community. Gandhi said he did not regard flesh food necessary at any stage and wrote five books on vegetarianism. Gandhi wrote:

> I hold flesh-food to be unsuited to our species. We err in copying the lower animal world if we are superior to it.

Gandhi also wrote:

> The cow is a poem of pity, she is mother to millions of Indian mankind.

The Hindus see God in everything and in every form—trees and rivers, cows and even ants. They have reverence for life. This reverence is shown in the principle of "ahimsa." This is why most pious Hindus eat no meat because it would be against their religion to have an animal killed to provide them with food. The Scriptures warn,

> All that kill ... cows rot in hell for as many years as there are hairs on the body of the (slain) cow.

For a Hindu to eat beef is a sacrilege about equal to cannibalism. The wealthy men endow places to take care of old and decrepit cows and many Hindus bow deeply to all cows that they pass.

Even insects are protected by "ahimsa." A devout housewife will throw out crumbs as a gift of hospitality to the insects and on festival days she may put her rice flour before her doorway having made from it elaborate designs. These designs are good luck symbols that please the spirits who guard the doorway, but they also provide a banquet for the ants.

Throughout all of India's long history her people have depended upon cows and oxen for help. Pulling ploughs and carts, providing milk for drink and food and dung cakes for fuel in the homes, the cow has been India's most valued domestic animal,

In any Indian city it is startling to see traffic wait patiently while a cow ambles across the street. All are sacred animals and no loyal Hindu would bring harm to a cow. Their affection for the cow is unique and the worship of a cow is said to give a married woman sons. It is a worthy religious act to feed any wandering cow.

There are many festivals scattered throughout the year in India and the animals are given a part in the celebration. Fancy designs are painted on Temple elephants and cows are bathed and their heads decorated in patterns of yellow and red. Hindus believe sacred animals should have a share in happy days (from *The World's Great Religions—Life*).

Animals are protected in other religions also. In a picture I saw recently of the philosopher LaoTzu, Father of Taoism, he is pictured astride an ox. The ox is a symbol of spiritual strength.

Playwright George Bernard Shaw became a vegetarian at age twenty-five and it was Shelley who opened his eyes to "the savagery of my diet." When people told him that he looked youthful, he said this was not so—that he looked his age. He said it was the other people who looked older than they are and what could you expect from people who eat corpses? Quoted in *Higher Taste: A Guide to Gourmet Vegetarian Eating*, Shaw wrote this poem:

> We pray on Sundays that we may have light
> To guide our footsteps on the path we tread;

We are sick of war, we don't want to fight,
And yet we gorge ourselves upon the dead.

He wrote this as a comment on violence and flesh-eating in human society.

H.G. Wells wrote against the slaughter houses in "A Modern Utopia" and Nobel-prize winning author Isaac Bashevis Singer became a vegetarian in 1962 at age fifty-eight. He said he was very sorry that he had waited so long and he finds vegetarianism quite compatible with his mystical variety of Judaism. He made statements I truly appreciate and that are powerful—of how we pray to God for mercy and justice while we continue to eat the flesh of animals that are slaughtered on our account. He states this is not consistent. The ethical consideration comes first, for him, even though he appreciates the health aspect of vegetarianism. He made this statement:

Even if eating flesh was actually shown to be good for you, I would certainly still not eat it.

Gandhi also believed that ethical principles are the basis for vegetarianism and not reasons of health. I, too, feel as these two men have expressed themselves. Singer became impatient with all the intellectual rationalizing for meat-eating and he said that various philosophers and religious leaders tried to convince their disciples and followers that animals are nothing more than machines without a soul, without feelings. But he goes on to state that if anyone who has ever lived with an animal—be it dog, a bird, or even a mouse—knows that this theory is a brazen lie, invented to justify cruelty (from *The Higher Taste*).

It is this very point of view that I have been trying to express through my deep sharings concerning my relationship with Rochester.

There are so many more statements that touch the soul and cause one to pray and consider the turning away from killing and flesh-eating.

Jean-Jacques Rousseau, mentioned earlier, also wrote among many of his writings this heart-breaking observation that is all truth:

> The animals you eat are not those who devour others; you do not eat the carnivorous beasts, you take them as your pattern. You only hunger for the sweet and gentle creatures which harm no one, which follow you, serve you, and are devoured by you as the reward of their service.

Thoreau whose writings have influenced me for the good in many areas of life has also written:

> No human being past the thoughtless age of boyhood, will wantonly murder any creature which holds its life by the same tenure that he does. *(Walden)*

He has also written in *Walden:*

> I once had a sparrow alight on my shoulder for a moment while I was hoeing in a village garden, and I felt that I was more distinguished by the circumstance than I should have been by any epaulet I could have worn.

Henry Beston (1888–1968), author of a beautiful book *The Outermost House* and a naturalist who once lived on the beach of Cape Cod year round in a little hut, wrote:

> We need another and a wiser and perhaps a more mystical concept of animals. We patronize them for their incompleteness, for their tragic fate of having taken form so far below ourselves, and therein we err and err greatly. For the animal shall not be measured by man. In a world older and more complete than ours, they move finished and complete, gifted with extensions of the senses we have lost or never attained, living by voices we shall never hear. They are not brethren, they are

not underlings. They are other nations, caught with ourselves in the net of life and time, fellow prisoners of the splendor and travail of the earth.

And can Christians not be caused to search their souls upon reading these words of other human beings who have answered the call within their souls to respect all life and not kill, torture and eat creatures that were put on this earth in our trust?

I have been reading for several years on this subject and can come to no other conclusion than I have. I have collected the quotations and thoughts of others in a special Commonplace Book of my own and I will continue to do so. I cannot tell you the sources of all that I have shared with you in this chapter except that the words came from my own collected ones and many of these came from *The Extended Circle: A Commonplace Book on Animal Rights* that I have mentioned earlier, and *The Higher Taste: A Guide to Gourmet Vegetarian Cooking,* and *Walden* by Henry David Thoreau.

I will close this chapter with the words once more of Isaac Bashevis Singer (1904–   ):

> I personally am very pessimistic about the hope that humanity's disregard for animals will end soon. I'm sometimes afraid that we are approaching an epoch when the hunting of human beings may become a sport. But it is good that there are some people who express a deep protest against the killing and torturing of the helpless, playing with their fears of death, enjoying their misery. Even if God nor nature sides with the killers, the vegetarian is saying: "I protest the ways of God and man." We may admire God's wisdom but we are not obliged to praise what seems to us His lack of mercy. It may be that somewhere the Almighty has an answer for what He is doing. It may be that one day we shall grasp His answer. But as long as we don't understand it, we shouldn't agree and we shouldn't flatter Him.

As long as human beings will go on shedding the blood of animals, there will never be any peace. There is only one little step from killing animals to creating gas chambers a la Hitler and concentration camps a la Stalin—all such deeds are done in the name of "Social Justice." There will be no justice as long as man will stand with a knife or with a gun and destroy those who are weaker than he is (from *Foreword to Vegetarianism, A Way of Life* by Dudley Geyo and *The Extended Circle: A Common Place Book of Animal Rights*).

These have been powerful words from the hearts of many human beings that I have included in this subject of vegetarianism. May they be used mightily to touch other hearts. But I have not included why I know and believe that to stop killing and eating all creatures is a deeply spiritual matter. That truth I learned through my own personal experiences, not just through these collected quotations and my extensive reading. And that is why my commitment to vegetarianism is irrevocable. I shall share my experiences now.

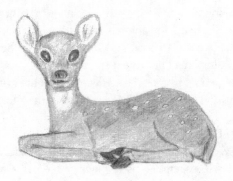

CHAPTER 5

The Commitment

"The only way to live is to live and let live."

—Mahatma K. Gandhi

"Thou shalt not kill."

—Exodus 20:13

On September 27, 1989 I became a vegetarian. Perhaps I should begin this testimony and statement by sharing "some" passages—not all—of that very simple journal entry I made regarding this.

New Hampshire

I am writing in green because it seems to represent nature and what I am about to enter has to do with nature. "Green is life" and this entry is about life—the life of animals and my life. From this moment on as I make this entry I am going to be a vegetarian. I will not eat meat of any kind, nor fish. I cannot let any living creature be killed for my sake that I might have food. I have not eaten red meat for many years and for a time gave up turkey and chicken. But always through family and circumstance and my own weakness, I went back to eating poultry. Though I cannot eat it after I prepare it myself and think it gross—and though I have given up preparing it, I can eat it in restaurants and at other's homes. This is wrong and I have been going against what I believe. I will also not eat fish, for fish are living creatures too.

I knew the health reasons for giving up all of these things due to studying the Macrobiotic Diet, but always I felt too, that it was wrong to kill animals for our food. Since Rochester has come into my life, the Lord has given me a deepening love for all creatures and sometimes to the point of tears. To think of them being slaughtered in horrendous ways drives me wild. I always wanted more spiritual evidence that this was wrong and yet others would say when it was discussed that animals were killed in the Bible, and men then ate meat etc.

I did not have evidence for what I felt personally. This has been growing in me for a long time. Suddenly last Saturday when at the book sale at the library and I was preparing to leave, I saw a book on the table called Higher Taste, and it was about the Vegetarian way of life. I took it, bought it, and once I began to read, in it I found the answers I have been searching for, and I was convicted in my spirit. I knew I could not now know what I do and continue to eat poultry and fish.

The scriptural evidence was there that I needed plus many other facts about cruelty to animals and their suffering, and the way our lives should be lived. I have been reading it each day and cannot go on as I was. I have to become a vegetarian and respect the lives of my fellow creatures.

Please, dear Jesus, give me strength to never go backwards even in the face of criticism or lack of understanding of family or friends. I must do as the Holy Spirit has led me to do. Shortly I will share this with Bob and I beg you to prepare his heart that he might understand. Thank you, dear Jesus. And I do this too, in deepest gratitude for the gift of Rochester in my life, who has a soul just as I have, and I want to honor him. Help me, dear Jesus. Thank you. Amen."

And I did share this with Bob, and through my prayers that preceded our discussion, he accepted my decision and commitment, and in time—a period of months—he joined me in the vegetarian way. Actually my commitment had been silently made in my heart September 26, the previous day, the 11th anniversary of my Mother's death. But we were en route to New Hampshire from Pennsylvania and spent most of the day in the van, and so I did not commit my commitment to writing until the following day, the twenty-seventh and made it official by my journal entry.

This segment of my spiritual journey actually traces back to 1983, when I read another book, which I can only describe in its affect on me as being almost comparable to having been confronted with Christ, in that I had to make a decision. I could not simply put the book aside when finished and go on as usual with my life. I had been given new knowledge that demanded a response and I responded in the only way my heart would let me. I said "yes." The book was *Recalled by Life* by Dr. Anthony Sattilaro, a Catholic physician who was head of Methodist Hospital in Philadelphia. It was his written testimony of being healed of cancer that was all through his body by adopting and living on the Macrobiotic Diet. I also identified with him because his life was changed in the summer of 1978 due to the diagnosis of his illness and the death of his father and the meeting of strangers who brought him the message of life with the news of this life-giving diet. My life too had been changed that same summer and into the fall just as his had, for I had the miracle given me that I could become a Catholic—a calling I had had in my soul for some years—followed by the death of my mother and then my actual reception into the Catholic Church. That the author also lived in Philadelphia was another tie. Shortly after completing the book, two of my daughters and I, along with many others we knew, were privileged to hear Dr. Sattilaro speak at a local Methodist Church. That night, in a deeply spiritual way, he shared his testimony in even more depth and showed before and after x-rays of his body—the before-ones filled with cancer and the after-ones revealing the absence of it. Following the talk he told many people in the audience illnesses and physical problems that existed in their bodies through the unusual method of Oriental diagnosis. This is the same method all Macrobiotic counsellors use when diagnosing conditions in people that come to them to be put on the Macrobiotic Diet for healing or prevention of illnesses. Many illnesses that Dr. Sattilaro diagnosed were confirmed right then to him by the people with him that they indeed had these conditions. Others were not aware that they had problems until he had told them; they were then advised to see their own physician concerning them.

This was an evening I have long remembered and I have reread his book at various times and given it to many others. He went on to write several more books and travelled all over the world to spread hope to others concerning the life-giving Macrobiotic Diet. Therefore, when learning the news last year that Dr. Sattilaro had died, I was deeply saddened and felt as if I had lost a friend. I do not know his cause of death, but even if cancer again appeared, he had been given twelve more years of life from his original diagnosis and cancer, and he used those twelve years to give hope and healing to countless others through his books and his travels and lectures. He left a legacy to all who will listen and we heard him tell that night in the Methodist Church of how his spiritual life had been deepened, and how he had been a fallen-away Catholic but had returned to the church and even to the attending of daily Mass and the reading of the Breviary.

I have written previously how my Macrobiotic cooking lessons helped others, for once I read *Recalled by Life*, I found a Macrobiotic Center and enrolled in the course. I only wish I had been more strict through the years, for though we still maintain the basics and eat in a vegetarian way, we do not eat a strict Macrobiotic Diet. But perhaps we shall come full circle and one day embrace it again, and in the meantime there is little of it that we are not using and always we have short grain brown rice and beans and vegetables. I feel privileged to have had Dr. Sattilaro and the Macrobiotic knowledge enter my life, and if I did it only for my dear little Peruvian friend Magdalena, it would have been worthwhile, for she was given two and a half years of life that she never could have had without it. She had been sent home from the hospital to die and I began to cook for her as did her daughter Martha—and later in Peru she was cared for in this way. There was nothing any physician could do for her, but the Great Physician opened my eyes to this diet through *Recalled by Life* and Magdalena's life was recalled for several more years. Praise God! It is our loss that we are not strict in it at the present, but that is now. Who is to say what will be? And I pray that readers will truly consider this way and read this powerful book by Dr. Sattilaro and see how Our Lord speaks to you through his writings. I hope your lives will be touched and changed as my life was. A fine explanation of this diet in a brief way is this one by Bill Tara:

> The diet which serves us best will be one which produces health and limits disease, is capable of being grown and produced by natural methods and produces adequate food for all the people of the world.

It does not involve the killing, torture and slaughtering of living creatures.

The name *Macrobiotics* is derived from the Greek, incidentally; "macro" means great, "bio" means vitality, and "biotics," the techniques of rejuvenation. I wish to say that in all my years of preparing meals for my large family it was during the period that I cooked strictly in the Macrobiotic way that I enjoyed cooking the most. I also found it most fulfilling because I knew I was giving the highest form of nourishment to my family. Even though the preparation of each meal took much longer than regular meal preparation of a normal diet, it was the happiest time of my life in regard to cooking. My finest advice to any reader at this point is to learn above all to cook rice and to cook it well—short grain organic brown rice. This is the type that is obtained in a health food store—not in a supermarket. This rice contains all the elements our bodies need and one can live on it exclusively as is proven. My husband and I did spend ten days on it alone and the benefits were incredible. But eating rice regularly would be a beginning for any reader into the vegetarian way. One does not have to be Macrobiotic. But brown rice should be in every Vegetarian diet and in every non-Vegetarian diet.

If it is a spiritual commitment to you and you are doing it as a moral act and for God and for the living creatures and not merely for a healthy diet, then you must be prepared and pray much. I have shared in great detail in a chapter in my book *Compassion for All Creatures* a testimony of what occurred in my life personally when I made this commitment. And I write these words now so that other readers might know and realize that it is no slight thing to murder, torture, slaughter, hunt and experiment on helpless animals. It is no slight matter when even one life is taken—human or creature. And my experience has been engraved on my soul and I know with all my being that it is immoral to murder another whose life you yourself can never replace. Therefore my life style and diet can never be responsible for another's death. My commitment is irrevocable as is my husband's, and I know it to be truth: "Thou shalt not kill"—not humans, not animals, not any living thing.

> "*If animals could talk, would we then dare to kill and eat them? How could we then justify such fratricide?*"
>
> —Francois Voltaire

May the Holy Spirit speak to your souls. The following poem was written October 15, 1989 following my commitment.

DO UNTO OTHERS

God in His Creation
Put upon this earth—

A host of marvelous animals
His Breath gave them their worth.

He did not want them slaughtered
He said "Thou shalt not kill"—
He wanted them to live in peace
Not at mercy of men's will.

He gave them woods and pastures
To live in nature's plan—
He did not want them tortured
By insensitivities of man.

He made them fellow creatures
In this universe so great,
They were not to fill men's bellies
And be sprawled across a plate!

Why must they kill such animals
As cow and lamb and pig—
Innocents cannot fight back
Oh men—you're not so big!

And what of jungle animals?
It is becoming clear—
Through senseless killings for great sport
Extinction comes—they disappear!

Do not justify these killings
Oh, you of human race—
Live and let live from this moment
Declare the end to this disgrace!

Close down the slaughter houses
Let the woods be hunter free—

Repent to God for all these lives—
And then a new world we will see.

In a somewhat lighter vein I add this poem written after Bob
answered an ad in a local New Hampshire newspaper and was
going to give me a gift of a lovely green leather sofa. It was like
new and a color we both admired. But I could not accept it and
as a result I wrote this in fun for Bob. How could I sit comfortably on such a sofa enjoying myself while writing a book of this
sort and having just made a spiritual commitment? Besides, the
lumpy old sofa had memories such as I have mentioned in a
previous chapter.

No, Thank You

It was a sofa that he tried
To give me—made of animal hide.
Made from a creature meant to roam—
And not to be inside our home.

It fit our needs so perfectly
And yet I had to disagree—
It could not come and fill the space—
Of older piece—now a disgrace.

A luxury, yes—and lovely green
But how compassionless, and mean
To add to slaughter of this cow
Deny commitments—weakly bow—

Just to have a sofa new
And own green leather soft, could you?
And he agreed with this—and now
Our sofa's still of lumps—not cow!

And this next poem, "The Commitment," was written on the second anniversary of this commitment—affirming anew that my decision is irrevocable. It is now twenty years and six months since I wrote the poem and I would not change a word.

THE COMMITMENT

Two years ago I did commit—
Stopped being then a hypocrite.
No longer could I say I care—
While eating creatures for my fare.
If animals I loved so dearly—
Then I had to say quite clearly,
That vegetarianism I'd embrace—
And not eat anything with a face.

Red meat I gave up long ago—
Dear lambs and cows I did forego.
All creatures in that category—
Became absolutely mandatory—
To exclude—I could not bear,
Their slaughter and the deep nightmare
That they endured so I might eat—
When eating meat is obsolete!

Suddenly I knew I could not—
Eat fish or poultry—no, I would not!
For they are creatures God gave life,
Not meant for strife and human knife—
But to survive—remain alive.
Can I as human—thrive, deprive,
A being of its right to live—
When there is known alternative?

I eat now beans and much brown rice;
Good fresh vegetables—perhaps a slice—
Of bread—and yes, spaghetti's nice—
It really is not sacrifice—
And yet each day I have a feast—
But not on fish or fowl or beast.
But now my soul does not protest.
For on my plate there is no guest!

And in these past years since this poem came into being, I have written dozens more about Rochester and all God's precious creatures. Some appear in my other books and others are just for myself alone written in my journals and notebooks. Perhaps you too would like to write poetry for your animal companions who inspire and comfort you, or for other creatures who may never have a poem written for them yet will know somehow in their hearts through His spirit that you have done this for them. It will give you a peace that passeth all understanding. I know. A poem I find very comforting, written by New Hampshire poet John Greenleaf Whittier, I often include in letters of sympathy and Mass cards. It is appropriate to write out in a letter to a friend grieving for an animal companion. It can be for all dear animals everywhere.

THE ANGEL OF PATIENCE

To weary hearts, to mourning homes,
God's meekest Angel gently comes.

No power has he to banish pain,
Or give us back our lost again;

And yet in tenderest love, our dear
And Heavenly Father sends him here.

There's quiet in that Angel's glance,
There's rest in his still countenance!

He mocks no grief with idle cheer,
Nor wounds with words the mourner's ear;

What ills and woes he may not cure
He kindly trains us to endure.

*"The animals you eat are not those who devour others; you do
not eat the carnivorous beasts, you take them as your pattern.
You only hunger for the sweet and gentle creatures which harm
no one, which follow you, serve you, and are devoured by you as
the reward of their service."*

—Jean-Jacques Rousseau

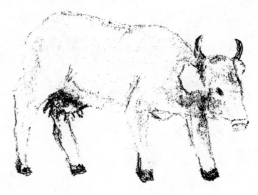

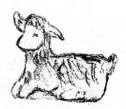
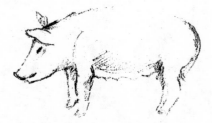

"*I have a friendly feeling towards pigs and consider them the most intelligent of beasts. I also like his attitudes towards all other creatures, especially man.*"

—W.H. Hudson, naturalist

CHAPTER 6

❖

Christian Thoughts on Animal Rights

"If we cut up beasts simply because they cannot prevent us and because we are backing our own side in the struggle for existence, it is only logical to cut up imbeciles, criminals, enemies, or capitalists for the same reason."

—C. S. Lewis, Christian Writer

AN INNER MORAL LAW should speak to the conscience of each Christian—that God's creatures should not be slaughtered, hunted and their flesh be eaten and worn for the pleasures of man when God has provided alternatives of worth in the world in the place of destroying sentient life.

As I began to collect quotations by Christians concerning the protection and saving of God's creatures from slaughter, torture, vivisection, experimentation and from being hunted, I became very disheartened. It was no easy work to find statements from Christians. In comparison to statements by those of other religions and by those whose religion was not stated but were humane individuals active in the Animal Rights Movement or in other societies in existence to protect and help all animals from those disasters I have listed above, the statements by Christians were in a tiny minority. I realize many Christians are involved in these active groups and are individuals that do their work of love and do not speak publicly about it. Nevertheless, despite that, there simply is not an abundance of support by Christians in the written word that would be a witness to all peoples of the world concerning God's Creatures and these terrible assaults upon their existence. One knows after reading about these issues where other religions stand. One knows the religions that protest killing and give compassion to all life—not just to human life. There is so much indifference and division about it amongst Christians that it is a very distressing situation. It is sad to know that Christians have the reputation for not caring and that because the Bible has stated that we have dominion over the animals that they then may be killed, eaten, tortured and all else that goes with these horrendous acts. There is little evidence that Christians in general believe that God's creatures were entrusted into our care and were meant to share the earth with us and to live out their natural lives, as humans may, if not beset by the similar violence that humans put upon the creatures. I point you to the book *Animal Liberation* by Peter Singer for an in-depth study of the word "dominion" and all things related to this. I am certain that if nothing else strikes the consciences of readers, the photographs alone in this book would cause any God-fearing believer to pause and search his own soul and experience a confrontation within. There are as well other quotations on these matters that are included in *The Extended Circle* edited by Jon Wynne Tyson.

The Views of Pope John Paul II

I will however include a quotation by Pope John Paul II that is in this chapter of "Man's Dominion" in *Animal Liberation* to show that a change is taking place and that the Pope urged that human development should include *"respect for the beings which constitute the natural world."* It is not an outright decree to stop the killing, as other religions have made and live by, but it was made as recently as 1988 and showed there was a definite change in the opposite direction, from a statement made by the Catholic Church in the second half of the twentieth century based on statements by Aquinas.

Pope John Paul II also added:

> The dominion granted to man by the Creator is not an absolute power, nor can one speak of a freedom to 'use and misuse' or to dispose of things as one pleases... When it comes to the natural world, we subject not only to biological laws, but also to moral ones, which cannot be violated with impunity (Encyclical *Solicitudeo Rei Socialis*, "On Social Concerns" from *Animal Liberation*, Peter Singer).

St. Thomas Aquinas, on the other hand, did not believe it was a sin to be cruel to animals and he stated we must not show any charity to them either. He believed it did not matter how man behaved toward animals and the statement made by the church in the second part of the twentieth century was based on Aquinas's thoughts and quoted from his statements.

Though I consider it a miracle through prayer and a blessing that I am a Catholic, I cannot agree with any part of this statement by Aquinas and simply am in shock that such a great thinker and theologian could come to such conclusions without his conscience being stricken. There have, however, been many humane Catholics—St. Francis of Assisi the exception most remembered. The wonderful St. Martin de Torres of Lima, Peru is another remembered for his love, care and protection of animals and for his many other Holy attributes. And there are humane Catholics in the world today who would not harm animals or consume them. I have mentioned other Saints in the past in this book who spoke out in defense of the animals.

The Example of Albert Schweitzer

This chapter would not be complete without mention of Albert Schweitzer, one of the twentieth century's greatest men. His book, *Out of My Life and Thought*, should be read by every Christian—and non-Christian also. To give him only a small part of a chapter when he deserves an entire book is sad, but one must really read for himself the book he has written rather than all I could relate about him here. Dr. Schweitzer speaks of Reverence for Life—he lived by this and states that:

> The idea of Reverence for Life offers itself as the realistic answer to the realistic question of how man and the world are related to each other.

He goes on to state, powerfully:

> As a being in an active relation to the world he comes into a spiritual relation with it by not living for himself alone, but feeling himself one with all life that comes within his reach.... Let a man once begin to think about the mystery of his life and the links which connect him with the life that fills the world, and he cannot but bring to bear upon his own life and all other life that comes within his reach the principle of Reverence for Life, and manifest this principal by ethical affirmation of life. Existence will thereby become harder for him in every respect than it would if he lived for himself, but at the same time it will be richer, more beautiful, and happier. It will become, instead of mere living, a real experience of life.... The ethic of Reverence for Life is the ethic of Love widened into universality. It is the ethic of Jesus, now recognized as a logical consequence of thought.

There are other words we must hear from him in this chapter for these words are from a man whose Lord was Jesus Christ.

The ethic of Reverence for Life is found particularly strange because it establishes no dividing line between higher and lower, between more valuable and less valuable life.... To the man who is truly ethical, all life is sacred, including that which from the human point of view seems lower in the scale.

Much more follows these writings of his just in one chapter alone of his book, but I will only attempt to share what spoke to my own heart in a powerful way and suggest once more that you read his wonderful book on your own. He states:

Devoted as I was from boyhood to the cause of the protection of animal life, it is a special joy to me that the universal ethic of Reverence for Life shows the sympathy with animals which is so often represented as sentimentality, to be a duty which no thinking man can escape.... When will the time come when public opinion will tolerate no longer any popular amusements which depend on the ill-treatment of animals!

And then to conclude these quotations of Dr. Schweitzer's I will include:

Christianity has need of thought that it may come to the consciousness of its real self. For centuries it treasured the great commandment of love and mercy as traditional truth without recognizing it as a reason for opposing slavery, witch burning, torture, and all the other ancient and medieval forms of inhumanity.... What Christianity needs is that it shall be filled to overflowing with the spirit of Jesus, and in the strength of that shall spiritualize itself into a living religion of inwardness and love. Only as such can it become the leaven in the spiritual life of mankind. Because I am devoted to Christianity in deep affection, I am trying to serve it with loyalty and sincerity.

In closing this portion on Dr. Schweitzer I would like to include these journal entries of Dr. Emory Ross of the Foreign

Missions Conference, who was the secretary-treasurer of The Albert Schweitzer Fellowship in America at the time he and his wife were at Lambarene in August 1946. They had arrived after dark, in the blackness of night and were greeted enthusiastically by Dr. Schweitzer—and Dr. Ross writes:

> Thus it was that we met this man whom we have always considered great, but whose true greatness was to grow and impress itself upon us in the few days we were privileged to spend in his presence, and in the presence of the work which he has hewn out of one of Africa's most jungled forests.

But it is this next entry in his journal that will show that Albert Schweitzer truly lived by the principle of Reverence for Life.

> At 7:30 the bell rang for breakfast, and we came out into the strange world which darkness had covered, as we came into it the night before. And what a world! Under the house and around it, is a veritable menagerie: Chickens, geese, turkeys, cats, dogs, goats, antelope, birds etc. A pelican is a faithful devotee and, although Mrs. Schweitzer insists on its going off to sleep, still it comes back daily to mingle with the congregation of birds and beasts which have gathered around Dr. Schweitzer—He is truly another St. Francis of Assisi. Nights, as he writes on his philosophy, a yellow and white cat which he saved as a kitten, curls up around his lamp. As he talked to us of Karl Barth and other philosophers he would occasionally stroke the cat's head tenderly and speak to it or of it.

In another book written about Dr. Schweitzer by Charles R. Jay, this same cat was mentioned and seen in a picture with the Doctor. The cat was on his desk as he worked and wrote prescriptions. Under the picture it was written that Sizi the cat often falls to sleep on the Doctor's left arm. The Doctor continues to write with his right hand, but he will not move his left arm while the cat is asleep on it.

Dr. Schweitzer remained at Lambarene without vacation for nearly ten years. Truly this is a great Christian man and one whom we cannot ignore in our spiritual journey to the principle of Reverence for Life. From out of his life and thoughts may we be helped and inspired to live in this humane way—for there is no other way if we are followers of Jesus—for it is an ethic of Love.

It becomes more and more evident that a clear and definite statement or creed concerning our fellow creatures who share this earth with us should be prayerfully promoted for consideration and that all Christian denominations should take part in the creating of it—and then in one Voice, Christians should tell the world their creed and forever stand by it. Ahimsa (harmlessness, non violence) is not just for other religions. It should be especially for Christians who claim to follow the One who is all Love.

I will close this chapter with a powerful statement by a Catholic Christian of this present time—who emphasized all I have tried to express and with whom I absolutely agree.

I am a Catholic and consequently for me there can be no vicarious satisfaction in the thought that a person who has misbehaved cruelly towards animals will pay for it in a future life, when he or she becomes a fox and is hunted by the very pack of which he (or she) was the proud master. It is clear to me, however that when, if ever, humanity lays aside its suicidal quarrels, and becomes one, the philosophical principle of Buddhism or Hinduism, in their attitude towards animals, must be integrated to the Way, the Truth and the Life of all mankind.

The so-called acceptance of natural cruelty as something over which we should shrug our shoulders is not the view which the purest religious thinkers have taken. To them cruelty is always cruelty and a hard thing, if not impossible to reconcile with the character of the All-Good.

It is our duty as men and women of God's redeemed creation to try not to increase the suffering of the world, but to lessen it. (Leslie G. Pine, 1907–)

May this speak to the hearts of all Christians.

CHAPTER 7

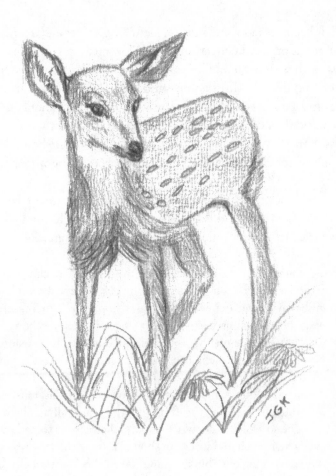

Closing Meditation

"There is not an animal on the earth, not a flying creature on two wings, but they are people like unto you."

—The Koran

"Be not forgetful to entertain strangers; for thereby some have entertained angels unawares. Remember them that are in bonds, as bound with them; and them which suffer adversity, as being yourselves also in body."

—Hebrews 13.2, 3 (K.J.V.)

"The greatness of a nation and its moral progress can be judged by the way its animals are treated."

—M. Gandhi

"I'm holding this cat in my arms so it can sleep, and what more is there."

—Hugh Prather

THE STILL SMALL VOICE

Within my heart I often grieve—
For there are many who believe,

That all God's creatures who are dumb—
To pain and cruelty—must be numb!

They do not know that in the glance
Of speechless animal—there by chance—
If time is taken—soul of the wise
Can understand and recognize—
A discourse splendid and from God—
In silent eyes of those who trod
And share this earth with human creatures—
And that dear dumb ones are His teachers.

If these words that are here penned
One simply cannot comprehend—
Then condescend to please befriend—
And to His Creatures love extend.
Two souls will then know still discourse—
From animal to human—with God as source.

Dedicated to all God's Creatures   Janice Gray Kolb

"The Star Thrower," a true account written by the well known writer, poet and anthropologist, Loren Eiseley—forever comes back to haunt one's mind and heart once it has been read. At least this has been so in the affect it has had on me, and it must be so concerning others, for the story has been quoted and rewritten in other books and spiritual magazines. It was originally told in so moving a way. I would like to share it now also, for it is worthy to read many times.

At dawn on a beach in Costabel there was a man walking. The beaches there, claims the writer, are littered with the debris of life that the sea rejects. Though they try, they cannot fight their way home through this surf. Repeatedly they are cast back upon the shore. The starfish are among those that are washed up and their tiny breathing pores are stuffed with sand. To an observer, it would seem that the night sky had showered them down and the long-limbed starfish were everywhere on the beaches as far as the eye could see. As the writer, walking along the beach, rounded the next point—he spotted a human figure in the distance and he said he had the posture of a god. It was a young man, and the writer noticed he was picking up starfish and flinging them into the sea. He questioned the youth when he finally caught up and stood by his side—as to why he was doing this. He answered that if they were left in the morning sun the stranded starfish would die. Though the beaches went on for miles and there were millions of starfish, this young man was performing the daily task of love by rescuing as many as he could.

Perhaps there are those who would think him ridiculous to believe his effort could make a difference, but to each starfish in the young boy's hand that he flung to safety in the waves, it truly did make a difference. On our journey through life there will be many starfish on our paths and how we meet them and treat them and respond can make a deep difference in our spiritual growth.

Recently in thinking and praying about all of this and quietly and deeply reflecting on it all, there seemed to be something unusual come to mind and break through into these sad moments—for any time I think of harm coming to animals in any form it is deep sadness to me. I do not know if it was the Holy Spirit speaking to me or just an insight that surfaced from the depths of my being, but it came to me forcibly that perhaps we, who hope and long to one day be accepted into Heaven and be given eternal life and then are welcomed into "this place" we await, may find an alarming surprise there.

Heavenly Princes in Disguise

Most of our lives we have been aware of Fairy Tales and beautifully created Disney movies made from such stories—of creatures or animals coming into contact with humans. If only a chosen human will give help in some specific way, the specific creature will be set free from a wicked spell and be turned back into his original form of handsome human. Two well-known tales of this sort are "The Frog Prince" and "Beauty and the Beast." There are others too that are not as well known as these. The magic of love given to the creatures in predesignated ways brings a transformation. Behold, there stands a human, no longer a frog or a beast!

The insight I had was just this. What if all the creatures God puts into our care here on earth are truly His charmed ones, His princes, His royalty set upon earth to see if we humans are capable of giving them true love, love so endearing that our spirits will mingle with theirs (which they do) thereby transforming them. Then, when we arrive in Heaven we will recognize in spirit precious animal companions, who will now be just as we—equal, not beneath us as many humans thought.

What if these precious animals, that are being slaughtered, hunted, abandoned, experimented upon and being subjected to every known horror including vivisection, will one day no longer be frogs and beasts or cats and dogs and lambs and cows to abuse, but will have dropped these outer garments and be creatures of light and beauty, belonging to Him? They will be shown to us then as having been the glorious means for us when they were on earth to advance in spiritual holiness and in the life of self-giving and deep Christian love. And what if we fail? What if those ones we show indifference to or despise or treat in horrendous ways are really divine beings in disguise but we do not want *"to do unto the least of these."* What if this be so? Please think upon this seriously!

Anyone who has ever had a deep relationship with an animal or has one now has frequently experienced times when something exists between animal and human that defies explanation—from a dimension not known. And that experience may be often repeated but never is less awesome. There comes the distinct feeling, an impression on one's soul, that a being or entity lives within the creature that seems human or divine. I personally have known this repeatedly with my Rochester. It continues to happen as we share our lives. There were moments I specifically remember with one little dog of mine, Lizzie, and most certainly with Katie, Jessica's dog.

Smile or laugh if you will, but those who have experienced it will not. They will understand what I am saying. Therefore, if there be even the slightest chance that these impressions I have been given in prayer and quietness and solitude are even bordering on the possible, can we risk doing anything to our animal friends that we would not want done to ourselves? Or can we risk indifference and not actively do something to ease their situations and make efforts to protect them and stop the killing?

Are we ready, truly ready to meet our Lord, or do we have some serious rethinking and prayer to do? Can we allow our senses and souls to be dulled?

Are we ready to meet not only our Lord—but the animals too that have passed into contact with us in small or large ways— or even the ones that did not that we never gave a thought or prayed for in their plights as if they did not exist or were not suffering? Are we in need of confession and forgiveness? Of repentance?

Perhaps, in our pondering we will be overwhelmingly grateful to still be on earth and have a second chance in regard to the way we view and take a stand for animals and birds and fish of creation. Perhaps we will know deep in our spirits that the God who breathed breath into us—breathed that same breath into His creatures and we are ALL God's creatures. One group should never cause the other group pain and suffering and death.

Please pray, and think on these things and forevermore be released from *"The Ostrich Syndrome."* It is written *"Thou shalt not kill."* There are other forms of killing in addition to the physical. There is horrendous cruelty in emotional and psychological "slayings."

If we can repeat the Golden Rule (Matthew 7:1 2) from scripture, *"Do unto others as we would have them do unto us"* (and every religion has its equivalent of the Golden Rule in its teachings), and know that we truly follow this in regard to our animals and creatures, as well as to humans, then Our Lord surely must be pleased. But if we cannot, are we truly ready to meet our Maker?

I include in closing a prayer Bob wrote for us a number of years ago adapted from an old one we recited as children and far more comforting. I have included it in each of my books except the first, and will again now in this one for you. Rochester was and is always included in this prayer—and in the palm of my hand rests his soft little white paws.

> *As I lay down to sleep this night,*
> *please keep me safe 'til morning light.*
> *Grant me sleep and needed rest,*
> *and fill my dreams with happiness.*
> *For Lord I know that with You near,*
> *there's nothing that I have to fear.*
> *Guide me where You want to lead,*
> *and be with those I love and need.*

Pray daily and ask God to speak to your soul concerning your personal path, which will lead you closer to His creatures in love and concern and protection.

Learn to look at His creatures in a new way. Ask to be shown in prayer what you can do to make His earth a safe and humane place for His animals to exist. Pray for their welfare, and in doing this I believe He will reveal to you your own special way for changing things in this world to help stop horrendous acts against animals, so that they, too, can live out their individual lives, just as you hope to continue to live out yours. To excuse yourself from even trying is the same as allowing them to be tortured and slain. You may not do the actual despicable acts and killings, but neither are you doing one thing to stop them! It is one and the same. Apathy and indifference are the killers just as much as the slaughterers. Albert Schweitzer has said, *"The quiet conscience is an invention of the devil."* Whose ambassadors are we in this world? God's or the devil's? Remember, *the same Breath that Breathed life into you Breathed it also into His creatures.* That fact alone should confront each soul in a collision impact and never again permit anyone to disregard another life—be it human or of another species. To say you would never harm an animal yet allow atrocities to continue against them is not of God. No being likes to suffer.

Therefore, do not inflict suffering either directly or through your own fears or apathy. *"Do unto others as you would have them do unto you,"* and remember the way of Ahimsa—that of non-violence.

A Remembrance in Memory of the One Who Led Me to Ahimsa

To the world he was just one
but to me he was the world.

—Unknown

i carry your heart with me (i carry it in my heart) i am never
without it (anywhere i go you go, my dear; and whatever is done by
only me
is your doing —

—e. e. cummings

I WAS LED TO THE PATH OF AHIMSA by my beloved little cat Rochester. Had he not been sent to me by God I do not know if I would have been a vegetarian. As you have read, his entrance into my life and his constant presence changed me forever. And it was through our mutual love that I knew that I could not be as I was before. I had to follow the path of Ahimsa.

52

My Rochester entered Heaven suddenly March 8, 2002. He and I had only a day's warning that this had to be. Just as his entrance into my life changed me forever and for good, so did his passing utterly change me. I have never been the same and would not want to be. I live in the sacrament of the moment and continue to share life with Rochester in spirit. We write books also as we always did since he first entered my life, so we may touch other lives with the message that is in his book. I close with a meditation from the first book written that followed his passing. There have been five other books that followed and there will be more. This meditation is from *In Corridors of Eternal Time: A Passage Through Grief—A Journal*

> *He had ceased to meet us in particular places*
> *in order to meet us everywhere.*
>
> —C.S. Lewis

Friday, June 21, 2002

The love I shared and still share forever with Rochester is a gift. I carry this grief gladly, for without it would mean I had never had Rochester in my life. It is a gift from our one life lived together. I cannot ever comprehend life without Rochester, and I would not trade one moment of this sorrow, even with all the pain, in contrast to never having lived and loved with Rochester. It was a spiritual dimension of living that defies explanation, and now it continues on still yet another plane until we are together in Heaven. Without Rochester I cannot imagine what the past almost sixteen years would have been.

Perhaps there are some who have lost human or animal companion loved ones, who wonder where their loved ones are. Please pray and find a peace in the certainty that they live on. I am secure in my belief of sharing life with Rochester in Heaven, and that my Dad is caring for him until I join them. Yet I know too, as many do, that my loved one is still here with me, for I experience him and sense him. His spirit never deserts me, never departs. He is around me, beside me, within me, and slumbers on my legs. This will always be so. It is an unfathomable comfort. It is a solace beyond words.

Losing my loved one's physical presence changed me. I see the world differently, and a sense of solid individualism has strengthened me. I do not have to answer to others about my grief. I am changed internally, spiritually, and in mysterious ways. There is a new person within that has stronger beliefs and an endurance level I did not know was ever possible. I believe Rochester's Anima, his breath and soul within me, his eternal gift to me, is this underlying strength. And yes, God's grace, and His Holy Spirit bestowed on me at conception. I have resources and power within me that rise up and sustain even in my most anguished moments of depletion, and of experiencing Rochester's physical absence. I believe it is my most devastating loss, yet I know it is imparting a wisdom to carry me through what days of my life I have left until I am in Heaven with Rochester. The life we had together cannot be duplicated. It was and is a divine gift. Both Rochester and I are transformed. You who read may come to know this transformation too, if you are deeply grieving for one who was and is a special world unto itself for you alone.

EVERYWHERE

He is near
My little dear—
He is far
He is my Star.

He is without He is within—
In the silence
In the din.

He sustains
He ordains—
Removes fear
He is here.

For eternal   JGK
Rochester

Another Friday. Another Holy Hour from 5 to 6 PM in solitude, remembrance, prayer, tears, and eternal love. He is here.

The life we had together cannot be duplicated. It was and is a divine gift.

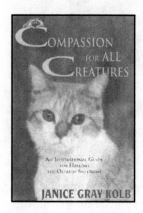

Rochester on the cover of the book he inspired—as well as the lifestyle of vegetarianism

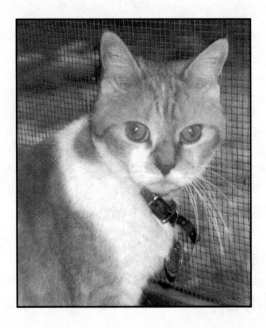

Rochester, beloved feline companion, confidant, counsellor, and ministering angel, finished his work here after almost sixteen years (minus one month), and passed on. He was a motivator and enabler to me and unselfishly gave of himself in deep love continually. He was with me every day—all day while I wrote, since he was eight weeks old, and was my inspiration. He was with me through every night. Rochester was the Star of every book I wrote. He was most loving friend to Bob. His sudden illness diagnosed only Thursday, March 7th brought about his reluctant departure. We were with him 'til he passed—and after. He shall forever be with me in soul and spirit, to help and inspire until we are together once more.

Rochester entered Heaven
March 8, 2002
5:07 PM

A *Remembrance*

Life-like 5x7 portrait of Rochester created by artist Tom Peterson, a gift from Tom and Sue Peterson from Colorado, that arrived the very day that Rochester's book *In Corridors of Eternal Time* was finalized. It appears also in *Solace of Solitude*, *A Pilgrim on Life's Road*, *Cherishing*, *Silent Keepers* and *Reflections by the Lake*. This portrait has been drawn by a loving man I have never met and came to me in a handsome frame. How precious my friends have created such a gift for me. It indicates too the power of love and inspiration my Rochester causes to emanate to others. Tom and Sue have many beloved animal companions of their own and extend help to other animals in many ways. Rochester introduced us through Sue's reading of my *Journal of Love*.

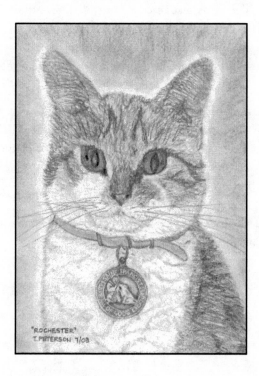

MY SELLA*

The shadow of my soul—my heart
Is a soft and furry counterpart
Of all I am and feel and think—
And a most mysterious link
With God. A consecrated connection
Sent by Him, a perfection
Of love and joy, one who is always there
Waiting to follow. Such a pair
My Sella and I—for we
Are bonded spiritually—
One in Him—God drew no line.
My Sella, My Shadow—is divine—
And overshadows me in comprehending
The unseen realm. In gratitude for sending
This gift of playfulness, peace and protection—
I pause daily in awe and reflection
Upon this inseparable companion—this life force—
And I humbly thank Him—our Source.

Dedicated to
my Rochester—my Sella
with love
in the estimated
month of his birth

JGK
April 10, 1996
New Hampshire

* Sella means Shadow. Taken from the poem by that name written by
William Cullen Bryant

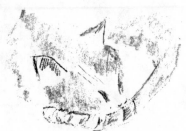

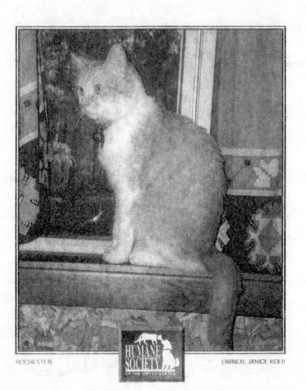

ROCHESTER   OWNER: JANICE KOLB

Picture of Rochester as he appears in the Humane Society of America's Desk Calendar for 1996. In the accompanying letter of congratulations it stated that he was chosen from over 20,000 entries. I have always had Thanksgiving in my heart for him in my life—so I was deeply moved to learn his picture appears on Thanksgiving Day—November 28, 1996. I had wished to honor him and entered his photo in the contest.

—JGK

ALL GOD'S CREATURES

by Robert A. Kolb Jr.

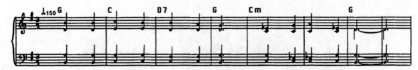

(1) All God's creatures have some rights—Man and Beast and Fowl.
(2) If we call Him Father God—then it must be true.
(3) How can we without a thought—say the "Golden Rule"
(4) All God's Creatures have more rights—than just live and die.
(5) Man's dominion doesn't mean—he must subjugate.

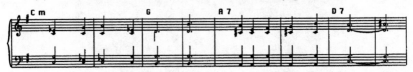

(1) Every little sparrow—each fox and every cow.
(2) That we're surely brothers—to things He Fathered too.
(3) Then abuse God's creatures—willfully be so cruel.
(4) We are often heartless—don't even really try.
(5) All God's precious creatures—should man control their fate?

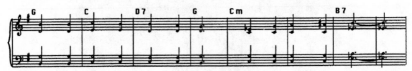

(1) All are part of His Great Plan—for he loves us all.
(2) For He blew the breath of life—into every breast.
(3) Oft' compassion is ignored—we should turn in shame.
(4) We sit back and then pretend—that we do not see.
(5) There's responsibility—not just selfish gain.

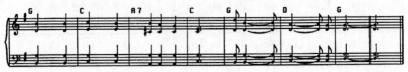

(1) If we love Him then we must love—creatures Great and Small.
(2) Placed a spirit deep down inside—and all creatures blessed.
(3) From the least—the last—and the lost—from the sick and lame.
(4) God's dear face and hear His strong voice—"Let my creatures free!"
(5) And compassion for all of life—and all creatures' pain.

Declaration of the Rights of Animals

Whereas it is self-evident

That we share the earth with other creatures, great and small.

That many of these animals experience pleasure and pain,

That these animals deserve our just treatment and

That these animals are unable to speak for themselves,

We do therefore declare that these animals

Have the right to live free from human exploitation, whether in name of science or sport, exhibition or service, food or fashion;

Have the right to live in harmony with their nature rather than according to human desires;

Have the right to live on a healthy planet.

    This declaration on animal rights was proclaimed and adopted by the 30,000 participants in the March for the Animals in Washington. DC on June 10, 1990.

—from *The Animal Rights Handbook:*
Everyday Ways to Save Animal Lives

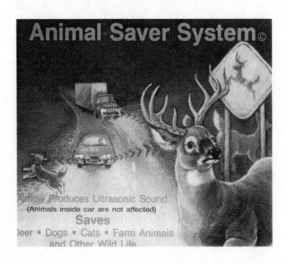

Advertisement for Wildlife Siren

This product can be purchased to put on the outside of your car. Once attached in an inconspicuous place it is activated by the passage of air through it and will help save the lives of all creatures and wildlife.

The Moose on the Cover

*"One does not meet oneself until one catches
the reflection from an eye other than human."*
—Loren Eisely from *The Unexpected Universe*

I FOUND THE WONDER of this statement by Loren Eisely a number of years ago when a large female moose chose to spend two weeks on our property. New Hampshire is Moose Country with signs on roads that read "Moose Crossing" and "Brake for Moose." So when I see a moose strapped to the top of a car or in the back of a truck during the hunting season allowed for them, it is heartbreaking. On national TV news we see people proud to have killed a moose and the personal reward of being able to eat Mooseburgers.

One specific day I spent many hours alone with this moose in a wooded area near our cottage during the two-week period she was here.

It is a period of time that has remained magical and other-worldly. Sometimes I would stand, and sometimes I would sit on the ground near her or on big fallen branches, but all the while I kept company with this beautiful moose we had named Matilda. While she ate branches, she would turn and look at me when I spoke to her and made me feel acknowledged. Never did she show aggression but just continued to eat and stroll and stay near me. She made no attempt to leave the wooded area in all the hours we shared. She could have charged past me but chose to remain.

That she elected to stay made me feel honored. I was in the company of a great mysterious creature. Though we had been looking at each other for hours, there came a moment so incredible when she slowly turned her massive head. Her big brown eyes stared deeply into mine at closer range. I stood motionless, held by her gaze. It was a moment of time so filled with the wonder of another realm.

She truly called me to another dimension in those hours spent alone with her. They were her gift to me. I felt it was a visitation, and she came to help me learn things I needed to know.

CLOSE ENCOUNTER WITH A MOOSE

She is chomping branches—
    and as I move in quietly,
        she compliantly
           allows my presence—
                with occasional glances
                    at this stranger.
As I gaze at the eloquence
    of this massive creature—
        and speak to her gently,
           I sense no danger.
I am a beseecher
    on behalf of the human race,
        as I intently
           speak love in this quiet place;
Revealing my respect—
    yearning to protect—

seeking to connect
with this wondrous teacher.

For Matilda   Jan
Moose of our woods

That anyone could stalk and deliberately kill these creatures of God for sport is beyond comprehension.

Reference Books for Further Reading

Abehsera, Michel. *Zen Macrobiotic Cooking* (Oriental and Traditional Recipes). New York: Avon Books, 1970.

The Animal Rights Handbook: Every Day Ways to Save Animal Lives. Venice, CA: Living Planet Press, 1990

Armory, Cleveland. *The Cat Who Came for Christmas.* Boston, Toronto, London: Little, Brown & Co., 1987.

Armory, Cleveland. *The Cat and the Curmudgeon.* Boston, Toronto, London: Little, Brown & Co., 1990.

Boone, J. Allen. *Kinship with All Life.* New York: Harper & Row, 1954, 1976.

Briggs, Anna C. *For the Love of Animals.* Potomac Publishing Co., 1990. (The story of the National Humane Education Society.)

Bustad, D.V.M., Ph.D., Leo K. *Compassion: Our Last Great Hope.* Selected speeches. Renton, WA: The Delta Society, 1990.

Camuti, Dr. Louis J. with Frankel, Marilyn & Haskel. *All My Patients Are Under the Bed.* New York: Simon & Schuster, 1980. (Memoirs of a cat doctor.)

Caras, Roger A. *A Cat Is Watching.* New York: Simon & Schuster, 1989. (A look at the way cats see us.)

Caras, Roger A. *The Cats of Thistle Hill—A Mostly Peaceable Kingdom.* New York: Simon & Schuster, 1994.

Diamond, Marilyn. *The American Vegetarian Cookbook*. New York: Warner Books, 1990.

Fox, Dr. Michael W. & Weintraub, Pamela. *You Can Save the Animals: 50 Things to Do Right Now*. New York: St. Martin's Press, 1991.

Frazier, Anita with Eckroate, Norma. *The Natural Cat: A Holistic Guide for Finicky Owners, Revised Edition*. New York: Dutton, 1981, 1983, 1991.

Gallico, Paul W. (Transl. from the Feline & Ed.) *The Silent Miaow*. New York: Crown Publishers, 1985.

George, Jean Craighead. *How to Talk to Your Cat*. New York: Warner Books, 1985. (Offers insight into animal communication. Also *How to Talk to Your Dog*.)

Herriot, James. *All Things Wise and Wonderful*. New York: St. Martins Press, 1977. (Also *All Things Bright and Beautiful*, *All Creatures Great and Small*, and other books.)

Jenkins, Peter. *Close Friends*. New York: William Morrow and Co., 1985. (Warm, loving memories of his most remarkable pets and companions. Author of best seller, *Walk Across America*, and others.)

Joy, Charles R. (Transl. & Ed.). *The Animal World of Albert Schweitzer: Jungle Insights into Reverence for Life*. Boston: Beacon Press, 1950, 1959.

Koller, Alice. *The Stations of Solitude*. New York: William Morrow and Co., 1990.

Kosins, Martin Scot. *Maya's First Rose (A Memoir of Undying Devotion for Anyone Who Has Ever Lost a Pet)*. New York: Berkley Publishing, 1992, 1994, 1996.

Kowalski, Gary. *The Souls of Animals*. Walpole, NH: Stillpoint Publishing, 1991.

Marshall, Bruce. *Thoughts of My Cats*. Boston: Houghton Mifflin, 1954.

Masson, Jeffrey Moussaieff & McCarthy, Susan. *When Elephants Weep: The Emotional Lives of Animals*. New York: Delacorte Press, 1995.

Morris, Desmond (author of *Catwatching, Dogwatching, Horse-watching, Catlore*, and others). *The Animal Contract*. London: Virgin Books, 1990.

Newkirk, Ingrid (National Director, People for the Ethical of Animals [PETA]). *Save the Animals: 101 Easy Things You Can Do*. New York: Warner Books, 1990.

Newkirk, Ingrid. *Kids Can Save the Animals! 101 Easy Things You Can Do*. New York: Warner Books, 1991.

Sattilaro, Dr. Anthony. *Recalled by Life*. Boston: Houghton Mifflin, 1982.

Schweitzer, Albert. *Out of My Life and Thought*. Baltimore, MD: Johns Hopkins University Press, 2009.

Sequoia, Anna. *67 Ways to Save the Animals*. New York: Harper-Collins. 1990.

Singer, Peter. *Animal Liberation*. New York: New York Review of Books, 1975, 1990. (Considered the "Bible" of the Animal Rights Movement.)

Singer, Peter (Ed.). *In Defense of Animals*. New York: Harper & Row, 1985.

Townsend, Irving (Collector). *Separate Lifetimes*. Exeter, NH: J.N. Townsend Pub., 1986, 1990.

Wynne-Tyson, Jon (Ed.). *The Extended Circle: A Commonplace Book of Animal Rights*. New York: Paragon House, 1955, 1989.

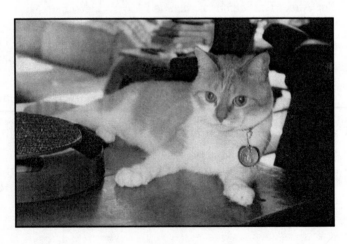

May I add still
a new book to tempt
you to try creating delicious Vegan
and Vegetarian meals.
It is published by my own publisher,
Blue Dolphin Publishing, and titled
Vegan Inspiration
Whole Food Recipes for Life
by Vegan chef Todd Dacy, with Jia Patton.

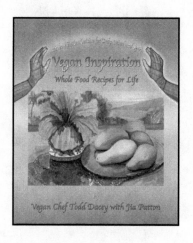

I am very pleased my own book,
*Compassion for All Creatures: An Inspirational
Guide for Healing the Ostrich Syndrome,*
is mentioned several times on these pages.

My beloved husband
Bob
entered heaven suddenly
April 3, 2011

He is eternally in my soul
until we are forever together
once more.

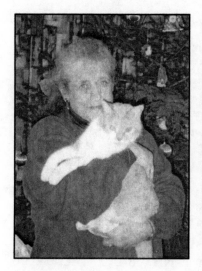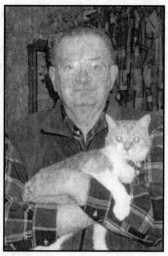

*J*anice Kolb, along with her husband Bob, are the parents of six grown children and have nineteen grandchildren and three great grandchildren. Their life has revolved around raising a loving family with religious values. In addition to raising their family, Janice developed a letter writing and audio tape ministry that gives encouragement and spiritual support to those who need it all over the United States.

Other inspirational works published by Janice Kolb include:
Higher Ground
Compassion for all Creatures
Journal of Love
The Enchantment of Writing
Beneath the Stars and Trees ... there is a place
Beside the Still Waters
Silent Violence
In Corridors of Eternal Time
Solace of Solitude
A Pilgrim on Life's Road

Cherishing
Silent Keepers
Reflections by the Lake
The Astonishing Adventures of Luki Tawdry

In a cooperative effort Janice wrote the book
Whispered Notes, with her husband Bob

Any correspondence to the author may be addressed to :
Janice Gray Kolb
P.O.Box 5
East Wakefield, NH 03830
jan@janicegraykolb.com

Visit her website at
www.janicegraykolb.com

Also by Janice Gray Kolb

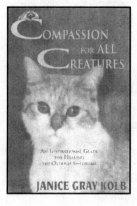

Compassion for All Creatures
An Inspirational Guide for Healing the Ostrich Syndrome
ISBN: 978-1-57733-008-0, 264 pp., 47 illus., 6x9, $12.95

A personal book of experiences, confessions, and deep thoughts praising all God's creatures through photos, poems and meditations. It is an impassioned voice for examining animal rights.

"Jan Kolb has written a very special book that will surprise you in many ways. Learning compassion and reverence by way of the animal kingdom makes perfect sense. She ponders deep questions and important issues which inspire her passion for all of life."
—Terry Lynn Taylor, *Messengers of Light*

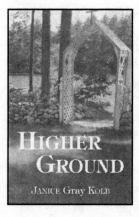

Higher Ground
ISBN: 978-1-57733-071-4, 176 pp., 16 illus., 5.75 x 8.75 hardcover, $14.95

Written from the heart, *Higher Ground* is a small treasure reserved for those who retreat into the silence and who wish to renew their purpose for living. It chronicles the experiences and thoughts of a woman on retreat in the woods of New Hampshire as she deals with personal fears and family problems and shares her faith.

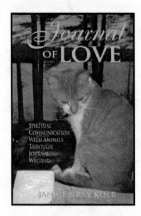

Journal of Love
Spiritual Communication with Animals Through Journal Writing
ISBN: 978-1-57733-046-2, 180 pp., 30 illus., 6x9, $14.95

Janice Kolb shares her heart-lifting journey of discovery as she learns to communicate with her beloved feline companion, Rochester—first by using her intuition and then by writing a journal of their "conversations."

"Once again the delightful and insightful Jan Kolb has provided all of us who truly love animals with another warm and wonderful book about how we may enter into deeper communication with our beloved pets."

—Brad Steiger & Sherry Hansen Steiger, *Animal Miracles*

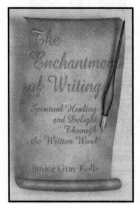

The Enchantment of Writing
Spiritual Healing and Delight Through the Written Word
ISBN: 978-1-57733-073-8, 312 pp., 48 illus., 6x9, $17.95

Janice Kolb shares events from her life that illustrate how to train yourself to write daily. Her encouragement and guidance for writing lead naturally to self-discovery. By preserving your thoughts and experiences, you discover new sources of guidance and insight.

"There are angels cheering for us when we lift up our pens, because they know we want to do it. In this torrential moment we have decided to change the energy of the world. We are going to write down what we think. Right or wrong doesn't matter. We are standing up and saying who we are."

—Natalie Goldberg from *Wild Mind*

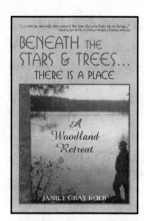

Beneath the Stars & Trees ... there is a place

A Woodland Retreat

ISBN: 978-1-57733-106-3, 372 pp., 47 illus., 6x9, $19.95

Beneath the Stars & Trees will help you withdraw from life's distractions and retreat to a place where you can see clearly the multitude of complex factors that make up your life. Share in thoughts and experiences which can open your mind to a world of peace and new possibilities for your life.

"Join Janice Kolb in a sometimes quirky, always perky, jaunt through lake-in-the-woods living, full of shapeshifting and kitty-cat angels, touching journal entries and frolicking poems, prayer chairs and little gnome tea parties—plus a spiritual encounter with a moose you're sure to remember forever."

—Michael Burnham, writer/journalist

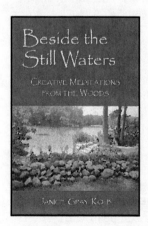

Beside the Still Waters

Creative Meditations from the Woods

ISBN: 978-1-57733-122-3, 276 pp., 11 illus., 6x9, $16.95

Beside the Still Waters is a personal view of prayer. Jan suggests a variety of ways to be in constant contact with God. These meditations can transform your prayer life into a source of personal fulfillment, power and strength. Many of these prayers may be familiar; others may be new to you. Being open to all that you read, you may discover new pathways to God and loving consolation. Though written from a Christian perspective, these prayers can be adapted to other traditions.

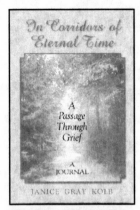

In Corridors of Eternal Time

A Passage Through Grief: A Journal

ISBN: 978-1-57733-135-3, 272 pp., 38 illus., 6x9, paperback, $16.95

The book is a passage through grief, written in journal form. It explores dreams, walking, memory loss, depression, examples of ways humans have grieved for humans, journal writing, and mourning a beloved companion.

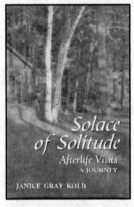

Solace of Solitude

Afterlife Visits: A Journey

ISBN: 978-1-57733-153-7, 300 pp., 6x9, paper, $17.95

This book was begun to find consolation after the sad events of 9/11. Then the death of Jan's beloved cat exposed her to a new view of life and death. She describes what she experienced and realized in solitude, which eventually brought solace.

A Pilgrim on Life's Road

Guidance for the Traveller:
A Continuing Journey

ISBN: 978-1-57733-176-6, 184 pp., 6x9, paper, $15.95

This is the last of the trilogy on grief and brings the author to the place where questions and aberrant thoughts have been dealt with. Grief has achieved a new dimension and now contains elements of resolution. The resolution of grief is not a single event, but a journey, which brings us to a place of sanity where growth can take place.